The **Positive Effects** of a **Health Care Manager** in **Women's Health**

by Dr. Patrice D Broderick

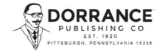

DORRANCE
PUBLISHING CO
EST. 1920
PITTSBURGH, PENNSYLVANIA 15238

Dorrance Publishing Co
585 Alpha Drive
Pittsburgh, PA 15238
Visit our website at *www.dorrancebookstore.com*

ISBN: 978-1-6386-7220-3
eISBN: 978-1-6386-7573-0

The **Positive Effects** of a **Health Care Manager** in **Women's Health**

Abstract

The study looks at the CDC reports and shows how the illnesses and diseases of women's health have not changed for 14 years. The study points out that the United States has come a long way, but we still have a long way to go. There have been many studies over the years, but there needs to be a new direction to solve the growing concern of women's healthcare. The issue has become a concern on a national level, which is evident with the passing of the Patient Protection Affordable Care Act (PPACA). The law entitles women to eight, no cost sharing preventive treatments. The study will look at the growing concern from the point of how the medical community can use preventive treatment of start changing the morbidity causes of death for women.

Keywords: Quality of Life, Morbidity, Healthcare, Lifetime, Cancer, standard of care, cost, Healthcare Manager, Doctor, Nurse

To my mother, Mrs. Jean Roberts-Smith,
and her two sisters, Carmen Govan and Ernestine Lewis.

Acknowledgements

I would like to thank my husband, children, and grandchildren for their love and patience during the time I was writing this manuscript. I would also like to thank all my professors at Colorado Technical University (CTU) for the encouragement. Also thank to Minister Doctor Black for her no-nonsense counseling and encouragement.

Table of Contents

Topic Overview/Background
Problem Opportunity Statement
Purpose Statement
Research Question(s)
Hypotheses/Propositions
Theoretical Perspectives/Conceptual Framework
Assumptions/Biases
Significance of the Study
Delimitations
Limitations
Definition of Terms
General Overview of the Research Design
Summary of Chapter One
Organization of Dissertation (or Proposal)

Review and Discussion of the Literature
(the exact headings will depend on the content)
Summary of Literature Review

Research Tradition(s)
Research Questions, Propositions, and/or Hypotheses
(as appropriate)
Research Design
Sampling Procedure

Instrumentation
Validity
Reliability
Data Collection
Data Analysis
Ethical Considerations
Summary of Chapter Three

Participant Demographics (if appropriate)
Presentation of the Data
Presentation and Discussion of Findings
Summary of Chapter Four

Findings and Conclusions
Limitations of the Study
Implications for Practice
Implications of Study and Recommendations for Future Research
Reflections
(as desired and authorized by the mentor and committee)

Chapter One

The study is about women's health. There have been many studies on women's health. They include topics like, "how do women feel about their doctors and health care?" They also cover topics about how illnesses affect women at different ages. There have been foundations, educational classes, and fundraising done for women on a national level. The problem is, the same top 10 morbidity issues have been the same since 1998. This is supported by the CDC reports of the top 10 morbidity concerns for women of all ages, (Leading Causes of Death by Age Females, All Females-United States 1998-2014). So why have they been the same? The research of articles is not because of a lack of concern or education. The study expands a phenomenology study that was done by Janette Perz and Jane M. Ussher on women who suffer from premenstrual syndrome. The study revealed that women don't only silence the self with premenstrual syndrome but with any illnesses.

A recent example of this would be the collapse of Secretary Clinton. She had a cough three days prior and made it seem unimportant during a speech she was giving. She never complained about the issues with her health care and it should not have reached the level of dehydration that caused her collapse. So the question is, why did she keep going and not say, "I am not feeling well"?

This type of reaction to illness is not just something that Secretary Clinton did but something all women do in the same situations (Cillizza, C. Sep 2013). The larger concern is the illnesses listed as one of the top 10 morbidity causes for women of all ages in the CDC (Leading Causes of Death by Age Females, All Females-United States 1998-2014). The study will also show how society and economics play a part in the concerns of women's health and how the recent healthcare law can help to make a difference in how social and the medical community treat and view women's healthcare.

Topic Overview/Background

Women still have many concerns when it comes to their health. There are several programs, like the Go Red Foundation that addresses one of the issues, but there is more than one pressing issue when it comes to women's health. Even though there is an awareness of the seriousness of women cardiovascular disease, some studies state it is still responsible for 29 percent of death in women reported to the CDC (Zamora, D, 2015). Cardiac Diseases are consistently in the number first, third, and fourth position of since 1998 in the Top 10 Morbidity concerns according to the CDC (Leading Causes of Death by Age Female, All Females-United States, 1998-2014). When a woman does not feel well, she realizes it. The issue is, will she take the time needed to take care of herself? The women who suffer in silence are considered to be a real female in our society. Placing the needs of others above her own is her ongoing sacrifice in life. So, many times, women will suffer in silence. She will never let you know the woman within (Perz, J. & Ussher, J. M., Nov 2006).

So, why is this a problem? Women's economic and social status has come a very long way, but women's health still needs to be overhauled.

The problems are not just for women, but the families and friends of the women. I watched this movie where a woman in her early fifties was diagnosed with early onset Alzheimer's. She had been to several appointments before she told her husband about her concerns. He thought it was just business as usual. My belief is the only reason she said anything to him was because her doctors asked her to bring someone with her. The first time she was supposed to ask him, she didn't. She said she did not feel it was necessary (Still Alice, 2014).

The illustration is what the suffering-in-silence wives, mothers, and professional business women represent today. Many doctors and other healthcare professionals are aware of the issue, but what is next step? How do they bridge the gap between what the women they reveal externally and what the women conceal? The healthcare community has a lot of growing to do when it comes to women's health concerns. The recent passing of the Patient Protection Affordable Care Act has a provision that includes no cost sharing preventive care for women.

Problem Statement

The problem to be addressed in the proposed study is women's health care programs in the medical community are not adequately supporting the needs of the women because strategies for identifying the early stages of women's diseases and illnesses have not been established (http://www.cdc.gov/nchs/deaths.htm, HHS, CDC, NCHS, 1998-2013). The research takes the approach from the theory of suffering in silence. Women are the caretakers of the world, and they suffer in silence and make daily sacrifices for their friends and families. The research study will examine this phenomenon and help to identify the possible solutions (Perz, J., & Ussher, J. M., Nov 2006).

Purpose Statement

The purpose of the proposed exploratory qualitative study is to explore the strategies for identifying the early stages of women's diseases and illnesses. Over the years, there have been several programs that support the betterment of women's health. Examples of these programs are The Go Red Foundation, whose goal is to bring attention to the women's health concern of heart disease and save lives (About Go Red, 2016), and Women's Cancer Fund Remembrance Run, whose mission is to help raise funds for patients while they are undergoing treatment (http://www.remberancerun.com/womens-cancer-fund, 2016). There are also other organizations like the Foundation for Women's Cancer, which is committed to widely sharing information about women's gynecological cancers (Other Resources, Foundation for Women's Cancer, 2016).

In this study, the top 10 morbidity health issues from 1998 to 2013 by age for all women will be examined (http://www.cdc.gov/nchs/deaths.htm, HHS, CDC, NCHS, 2016). The color chart at the end of the study will show the health concerns in the United States have remained the same for the last 14 years. The question is why some concerns are still in the top 10 positions after all the educational programs, foundations, and other resources for women that have been started. The high morbidity rate is a concern for healthcare in the United States. The concern for women's health has become such a high priority, it has been included as a major part of the new healthcare legislation that is called Patient Protect and Affordable Care Act, or PPACA (Sifferlin, A., Aug 1, 2012).

The fact that from 1998 to 2013 the same concerns are still so relevant that eight preventive treatments for women have been included the controversial healthcare act in our society today. The possible cause is being expanded in this study from more than one health issue to all illnesses and injuries. The study will take the direction of how can healthcare professionals become an active part of changing how women's healthcare is managed.

Research Question

The need for females to stop suffering in silence is the direction of the research study. Amending the continual morbidity issues of women in the United States is the primary focus of this study. The proposed research question of this study is as follows:

> **RQ:** What are the strategies for identifying the early stages of women's diseases and illnesses?

Propositions

The study is on women's health. Many studies have been done on education when it comes to women's health. There have also been many studies on the illnesses and disease that concern women. My research is centered on why, in our society, there is still high morbidity the same 10 conditions since 1998 (Leading Causes of Death by Age Group, All Females-United States, 1998-2013).

Conceptual Framework

The foundational framework of the study starts with the CDC reports. The phenomenon of silencing the self that was initially researched in November 2006 for women who suffer from premenstrual syndrome is the gap in the science. Since 1998, the same top 10 morbidity issues for women have been a concern. The sociology and economics of women will be explored as a matter that is related how we function in society. Then the issue will be brought up in recent years with the Patient Protection Affordable Care Act (PPACA) and the responsibilities of medical professionals under the new law.

Assumptions/Biases

The initial premise of the study was that women's medical issues continued because there was a lack of education. The second was the medical community has neglected women's health concerns and problems, and they needed to get their stuff together. Why has the medical community not done anything about the glaring issue so unresolved issues in women's health? These bias and assumptions were borne from experiences the researcher had at a medical processing site for National Guard and Reserve soldiers. Some of the doctors of all genders there made jokes about the lack of care and understanding of many of the women coming to the site. The researcher's mother passed away due to complication while being treated for ovarian cancer. The questions that were borne from this experience were, "How could the medical professionals that worked with her every day not see her symptoms? What was the doctor thinking, and how did she not notice the symptoms?"

Since starting this research, there has been a realization that no one was to blame for any of the reactions, lack of action, or understanding of either of these issues. The environment around us influences and supports both the attitudes for society's response to the medical concern and issues of women's health.

Significance of the Study

The importance of women's health has become a national issue. The proof of the statement is in the fact there is a special provision in one of the most controversial acts of our time. President Obama signed the Patient Protection and Affordable Care Act in March 2010. The provisions in this bill put into effect eight preventive care services that women can get without any cost sharing. Most of them are counseling, but we have tried everything else, so now it is time to talk (Sifferlin, A., Aug 1, 2012). The study is designed to change the role of the patient and the healthcare professionals. When a woman goes to the doctor, she knows just what she wants and decides which information she will take the time for following. An example is the recent healthcare scare of Secretary Clinton. Secretary Clinton's doctor recommended rest, but she chooses to continue to campaign (Cillizza, C., Sep 2013). This is not to say her choice was wrong, but the recent events may lead you to believe it was a dishonest decision. Influenza and pneumonia are number eight on the list of top 10 morbidity concerns of women in the United States of all ages (http://www.cdc.gov/nchs/deaths.htm, HHS, CDC, NCHS, 2016). Medical professionals need to take back control of the doctor's visit. Most experts know which women are going to listen and which are not going to listen. This study will show why it is important for them to take the next step that may save a life.

Delimitations

The possible overwhelming high level of importance of women's health at this time in our nation is something that will help but will also be an area concern. Many professionals and women will be interested in participating in the study. The focus of the survey is to find a way forward in changing the morbidity concerns of women in the United States.

Right now, you see women's health being covered on the news and a variety of talk shows. One of the programs that is unique to female concerns is the Dr. Oz Show. The show covers topics ranging from diet to reproduction (http://www.doctoroz.com, 2016). The recent collapse of Secretary Clinton was about women deciding to get it done. She agreed to campaign and not stop, and talked of her health. Like any woman at her level, her thought was to get it done and to do what she needed to take care of her professional responsibilities. She moved forward without complaint and presented a calm, put-together appearance. She downplayed several times her cough, and we all watched. She silenced the self and gave the appearance we all find acceptable. The actions of Secretary Clinton are a living example of the phenomenon that this research study is attempting to expand upon, not just one women's health concern, but all healthcare concerns of women in the United States (Perz. J. & Ussher, J. M., 2006). Even though there may be many healthcare professionals and females who would like to participate, the research survey will be limited to no more than 20 professionals and no less than 10 participants. There will also be no more than 10 essay questions. All the issues will be open-ended and will be designed so the participants will have to express their personal concerns.

Limitations

The boundaries of this study are the amount of time the participants will have to complete the survey. The next limitation is how many members will be willing to do a face-to-face interview (von Diether, B., 2016). The next is the scope. I have to keep the scope under control (Patterson, J., May 9, 2011). The topic of women's health is hot, but the goal is to examine how the healthcare community can develop a system to turn the issue around. It is evident from the study, women are going to continue to treat their healthcare with the same importance they always have because of their responsibilities of mothers and wives. Things that parallel the self-sacrificing behavior is also the way they show commitment to their work and business choices. The study takes the position that women need assistance with focusing on their healthcare, and who better than medical professionals to help?

Definition of Terms

Quality of life: A measurement that defines the real and negative aspects of a person's life. It could include where they live or their personal values and principles. For the purpose of this study, the best example is a measurement that gives a qualitative number to some years a person has to live if they have a chronic illness or if they are young (What is quality of life, 2016).

Morbidity: A state of being that is about an illness (Morbidity, Merriam Webster, 2016). For the purpose of this study, it is the lifespan of women who suffer from the top 10 illnesses as reported by the CDC.

Healthcare: The medical care provided to an individual by a person who is licensed to practice medicine (health care, 2016). For this study, it relates to the medical assistance given to women who have medical illnesses or injuries that affect their quality of life.

Standard of care: The quality of care that is provided to a patient (Definition of Standard of Care, 2016). For the purpose of this study, it relates to how women feel about the type of care they received. It is also linked to the quality of care their healthcare professionals feel they give.

Healthcare Manager: A person who ensures a medical facility is operating at its full capacity. They may also have to deal with the doctors and nurses to ensure they are meeting the standard of care expected for a patient in their care. For this study, a search will be done to identify the right type of healthcare manager to take part in a patient's care.

Doctor: A person who is licensed to practice medicine in different fields of medicine. For this study, it refers to those people who either practice medicine or physiology.

Nurse: A person who is a helper to the physicians who see patients. A nurse is a vital part of a patient's health care (Definition of Nursing, 2016). The roles of nurses have changed over the years; they are now responsible for entering information into the computer on patients that they did not have to do before. An example is they now check to ensure your medications are up to date and ask questions about your mental state of mind. For this study, it is related to their role as helpers to doctors who provide care for patients.

Patient Protection Affordable Care Act (PPACA): A new healthcare law that was enacted by President Obama in March of 2010. It will change the way insurance companies cover patients and extend care to patients who were not previously able to obtain coverage (Patient Protection and Affordable Care Act, 2016). For this study, it deals specifically with the eight preventive care services that are provided for women with no cost sharing.

Sociology: It is the study of a group of people and how they function in society. For the purpose of this study, it deals with how women operate in a patriarchal society.

Economics: Relating to person's ability to provide those things they need to survive. It can also be explained as the capacity to obtain and use the income they receive from their jobs to provide for their daily living expenses (Definition of economic, 2016). For this study, it deals with women and their ability to obtain the healthcare needed to support a high quality of life.

General Overview of the Research Design

The research design is a qualitative phenomenon study on women's health. The study will target the need for medical professionals to take control of the issue of women's health. It has become socially acceptable for the same top 10 illnesses and injuries to be a morbidity concern for females in the United States. The study will start with the review of CDC reports, sociology, and economics of women as it relates to their health. It also will speak to changes that the Patient Protection and Affordability Care Act have made on women's health. Then the final steps will be to get at the most 20 surveys with opened-ended questions and take those responses and project a possible way ahead for women's health.

Summary of Chapter One

Over the years, society has had foundations to help bring attention to women central concerns. The have been walks, talks, and organizations that are designed to assist women with medical concerns. The issue is, even with the walks, talks, and foundations, there have been the same top 10 morbidity concerns since 1998. Why, in the past years' medical advancements and help programs, this has not changed? The study expands upon a phenomenon called "silencing the self." The study also turns the spotlight onto medical professionals. Medical professionals have to take control the situation. What are their ideas of the way ahead for women's healthcare? Will the changes in the Patient Protection and Affordable Care Act have any effect on women's issues?

Organization of Dissertation

The reason this study is so important is that women's morbidity concerns have been the same for the last few years. Clearly, it is a concern because the most controversial act that has been passed in years included special provisions for women. The fact that eight, no cost sharing preventative treatments have been incorporated into recently the

Patient Protection and Affordability Act show that our leaders see the problem and want to make changes. The medical community needs to be evolved in this shift. The study gives them a chance to give thoughts on how they see this happening and how it can be successfully achieved. In chapter one, the foundation of the survey is briefed. Chapter two will cover the literature that supports the existence of the phenomenon. It will also include the lifestyle of women that many are contributing to the morbidity concerns. Chapter three covers how the research of the theory will be done.

Chapter Two

Our society is patriarchal, which means it is dominantly male over female (Giddens, Anthony, Duneier, M., Applebaum, R., & Carr, D., 2011). Looking at our society, you see women taking a back seat to men in the areas of decisions that concern women's issues. The reason for this is women are taught from youth that they need to avoid conflict at all cost; they need to protect themselves from failure; and they can never make mistakes (Bruce, J. May 13, 2016). They must be, at all times, calm and in control of their emotions. If they don't, then they are not what society accepts as a "good woman" (Perz, J., & Ussher, J. M., Nov 2006). They have the responsibility to take care of everyone in the family. Their husbands and children depend on them for everything. They are responsible for every aspect of their family's lives, and they must not fail. Over the years, there have been songs about women like "I'm Every Women," and "it's all in me." In the video from this song, you see the singer morph into several different women. Some jingles say, as women, you can bring home the bacon, fry it in a pan, and never let your husband forget he is a man. Then even in the historical, spiritual area, there is a Superwoman. She rises in the morning before dawn, ensures everyone in her family is fed, including the servants.

Then she proceeds to the docks to manage the family retail business. Once she is done, then she is off to the field to purchase land and make sure there is proper staff to operate the field in her absence. It may not be meant this way, but the whole time, this woman is running around town, working, while her husband is sitting at the local men's watering hole chatting it up with his friends. He is also doing it in the finest clothing. This is an acceptable picture, so we don't think anything of it, but it is an example of a patriarchy (Courtney, V., 2000).

Women are supposed to be efficient, untiring, and pleasantly dutiful at their entire task. Their families may not appreciate it, but in the case of the study done on the "virtuous women" by Vicki Courtney, the women are called blessed and praised by her family in the city they live (Courtney, V., 2000). In every example, you see women who can bring home the bacon, fry it up in a pan, and never let their husbands forget they are men. They are "every woman"; how else can they do all these tasks? From as far back as our society has been developing, women have carried the load. Yes, these days, we get to do a little roaring; but if we do too much, it is not taken well. The song "I Am Woman, Hear Me Roar" is a coming-of-age song that helped women develop a small voice. Yes, sisters are doing it for themselves these days, but it is not easy, and it comes at a price. Like "I'm Every Woman" mentioned above, both songs are examples of women's rights, but society doesn't like roaring women.

These types of examples of women are everywhere in our community. Even though a woman's primary purpose is still to be a helpmate to their husband and caregiver for their families, Superwoman and Wonder Woman are myths, we act as if these roles can be achieved by every woman in the world. Women in society do it differently now, but the standard is still the same Superwoman expectations. The only issue is, when we become ill or hurt, we never stop trying to be that Superwoman. In the lives of women, health concerns have emerged as a secondary concern until they cannot take the pain, or the symptoms get so bothersome, they want them to stop.

The above examples have often been used as descriptions of perfect women, wives, mothers, and virtuous women. In this description, there is nothing that says the woman suffers from the lack of sleep or exhaustion. In every example, her entire life is devoted to her husband, children, and household, even though in reality, women get tired or need time to rest after a hard day of work.

In a study done with ladies who suffer from premenstrual syndrome, it is stated that a real woman is one who is externally calm, in control, and self-sacrificing in relationships. It further describes the female reproductive body as the site of the monstrous feminine if a woman shows any anger or discomfort during the pain of premenstrual syndrome, (Perz, J. & Ussher, J. M., Nov 4, 2006). There was a scale used in this study called the "silencing the self" scale (STSS). Multiple subscales were developed in the survey called self-sacrifice, which measured women's ability to sacrifice their needs. Silencing the self is the measurement that describes the ability of women to express their opinions by avoiding conflict and possible loss of relationships. Two more scales that were used were 1) "externalized self-perception," which means judging the person by external standards; and 2) "divided self," which measures how well a woman shows an outer compliant self while becoming angry and hostile inside (Perz, J. & Ussher, J. M., Nov 2006). The study represented in this paper will take this further. The gap represented in this study will show that women not only use this form of self-denial when dealing with premenstrual syndrome, but every health condition they encounter. The study will further show how our society has accepted this concept that women who are externally calm, in control, and self-sacrificing in all their life experiences are thought to be the example of not just good women, but virtuous women (Courtney, V., 2000).

Women and Self-Sacrifice

A woman's desire to care for her family and present herself in a favorable light to bring respect and honor to her family will outweigh her need to take care of herself. We watch the same behavior play out day after day. A precise definition of silencing the self is a woman who has the outward appearance of a completely put together woman, who is always externally calm, in control of all her emotions, and never utters a word of complaint about anything, but the outward appearance is not the same as the woman inside. Inside, she could be in pain, angry, or unhappy with her a job circumstance, her intimate relationship, or even her relationship with her children. She could also not be feeling her best and dealing with a medical issue. The world will never know because, outside, she is the picture of perfection (Perz, J. & Ussher, J. M., Nov 2006).

An example of this would be two popular films that depict women who are ill but making sacrifices for their families. While watching these two movies, they showed the sacrifice of the women and responses to their illness was not noticeable the first time they were watched. After starting research on the phenomenon of silencing the self, the example of what society has come to accept is very clear. One movie was a movie called *Still Alice*. In the film a renowned professor is diagnosed with early on-set Alzheimer's. She has been directed to bring her husband to her next doctor's visit, but she does not because she does not think it's important enough to bother her husband. Other examples were the family members not noticing she had problems. When she and her husband finally shared the news of her condition and explained to her adult children that they needed to be tested for the gene, she was starting the later stages of the disease. Her oldest daughter found out she had the gene and, on a particularly rough day dealing with the disease, the professor wanted to run to her daughter's side to comfort her, (Nashawaty, C., Jan 23, 2015). Another movie is a comedy called *Tyler Perry's Big Happy Family*. When the woman's doctor tells her, her cancer is back, she tries to console the doctor by telling him there is not much he could have done. She also says to him she baked him his favorite cookies and not to worry; she understood he had done all he could. You laugh because it is supposed to be funny. The reality is, it is not funny. The sacrifice of this woman goes even further. She takes a bus across town and walks miles to her daughter's home to get help for her adopted son. The bad thing is, the daughter does not help her, and the adopted child is the daughter's child (Entertainment Weekly, Perry, T., Madea's Big Happy Family, Jan 21, 2001).

After starting the study, these scenes immediately came to the attention of the researcher. Like society, these women's behavior is thought to be acceptable and normal. Yes, the scene with the doctor was meant to lighten the mood and take away from the seriousness of the issues that are presented in the films. The behavior of these two women is not shocking. The influences of television, music, and even our historical backgrounds develop the "Superwoman" mentality that has supported the gap in the science the study is examining. All 10 of the top morbidity health concerns have remained the same since 1998. The problem could be the common consciousness of woman that silencing the self is normal and acceptable. They present one person on the outside while there is an entirely different woman inside. This is known as silencing the self or suffering in silence (Perz, J., & Ussher, J. M., Nov 2006),

Problem of Self-Sacrifice and Silence

The problem is that our society and women have accepted this behavior of self-sacrifice and used it as an example of a good and virtuous woman. So, now, my next question: Is silencing the self or self-sacrifice the reason why the top 10 morbidity health concerns have remained almost the same since the year of 1998? They may have taken turns in the fifth to eighth position, but they all remain the same (http://www.cdc.gov/nchs/deaths.htm, HHS, CDC, NCHS, 1998).

Dr. Flavia Bustreo, the Assistant Director-General for Family Women's and Children Health through the Life-Course, World Health Organization (WHO), stated in a speech in 2015 that we have come a long way, but we still have further to go (Bustreo, F., 2015). What did she mean by this statement? The top 10 women's health concerns we have as a nation are cancer, reproductive health, maternal health, HIV, sexually transmitted infections, violence against women, mental health, no communicable diseases, being young, and getting older. These issues are slightly different from those in the United States, but cancer and violence against women are still there on a national level. When you look at the CDC reports from 1998 to 2013 in the charts of this study, it will drive the concerns to the top of your awareness (http://www.cdc.gov/nchs/death.htm, 1998-2013). This is a significant fact and has become a concern of our government. The evidence of this is the Patient Protect and Affordability Care Act. Women's healthcare has become one of the new healthcare law's primary focuses (Di Venere, L., Sep 1, 2012).

Examination of Top 10 Concerns

Looking at the most recent report on CDC from 2013 shows the leading causes of death being heart disease, cancer, chronic lower respiratory disease, stroke, Alzheimer's, unintentional injuries, diabetes, influenza and pneumonia, kidney disease, and septicemia (http://www.cde.gov/nchs/death.htm HHS, CDC, NCHS, 2013). In 1998, the top 10 were the accidental and adverse effect, congenital anomalies, homicide, malignant neoplasms (cancer/tumors), heart disease, pneumonia and influenza, certain conditions originating in the prenatal period, septicemia, cardiovascular disease, and benign neoplasms (http://www.cdc.gov/nchs/death.htm HHS, CDC, NCHS, 1998).

In my complete study, I plan to add a chart with the years in between to better illustrate the similarity and movement of the illnesses and injuries. The silent suffering of women is a phenomenon that all ages of women are experiencing. It is considered a phenomenon because it is a natural psychological event that is happening naturally to a group of people (Giorgi, A., 2006). The method of phenomenology was first launched by Edmund Husserl, Martin Heidegger, Maurice Merleau-Ponty, and Jean-Paul Sartre. They explained it as a discipline that had its foundation of all philosophy (Stanford Encyclopedia of Philosophy, Dec 16, 2013). My study is a phenomenology study because as defined by these twentieth-century men. It is a study of consciousness as experienced from the first-person point of view (Stanford Encyclopedia of Philosophy, Dec 16, 2013). The "silence the self" consciousness is being experienced or lived by all women. They perform the state of consciousness naturally and suffer the consequences of the condition as a usual way of living (Stanford Encyclopedia of Philosophy, Dec 16, 2013). The topic of women's health has been studied over and over again from many points of view. The direction of the survey is one to identify the medical concerns, but once this is clarified, the research will take a difference approach and lean towards the management of these illnesses, diseases, and injuries. The study will collect data by using a qualitative approach. The reason for this approach is because the design of the survey is meant to give suggestions about a method of management that deals with how a group of people is experiencing a situation in their lives. It is also to offer suggestions about who in the medical community may be best suited to assist with the concern. The study will not be designed to prove or disprove anything. It is only intended to point out a possible gap in the science (Creswell, J. W., 2014).

The "silencing the self" event has become a way of life for women that can in many cases cause death. The reason it could end in the loss of life is that many women don't get help until it is too late to do anything about their condition. It has become a regularly accepted practice that is just thought of as a sad event. During the literature research process what has become evident is women are educated about their health, and they do care about it, but are still naturally placing it on the back burner when it comes to the roles and responsibilities they have in their lives. The research shows that they need help to manage the concern and to put it at the front of their consciousness before there can be a reduction in the morbidity levels of severe conditions, like cardiac disorders and cancer. For these reasons, a qualitative phenomenological study is the choice for this research project. The issue has gone on so long, it would be impossible for one study to find an answer to the problem in a matter of weeks. Every solution starts with a suggestion. That is the only desire for the study. Also, because the research leads to the outlook that the issue is a natural state of consciousness that it normal to our patriarchy, phenomenology is also the choice for the investigation process. The solution to the problem needs to lead back to the medical community. How can the healthcare community help? The first question for this study is:

> **RQ:** What processes can be put in place within the medical community to assist women to receive quality healthcare, and how might leaders of these organizations be held accountable?

Some examples of jobs in the healthcare community that can support would be physicians, nurse practitioners, nurses, or healthcare managers. Or will it take a team effort to help first acknowledge the concern and then develop practices that can help? Under the Patient Protection and Affordability Care Act (PPACA), healthcare managers have a deeper role when it comes to the management of patient care. Their roles have, in some cases, been expanded to the administration of physicians, nurse practitioners, and nurses. Depending on the size of the hospital, a clinic healthcare manager has duties that are ranging from the management of staff to the operation of the medical facility they work and overseeing the quality of care provided by their service (Lagace, M., 2016). The other essential responsibilities of doctors, nurses, and nurse practitioners have remained nearly the same. The only change is they must perform at a higher level of quality care or risk the hospital losing payment for a patient's care (ObamaCare and its Mandates Fact Sheet, 2016). The need to look into the additional roles of a healthcare manager and define the actual definition of their role in a medical facility is crucial to the validity of their role in the process of caring for patients.

An Overview of Healthcare Management

The role of a healthcare manager can mean many things. It depends on the size of the organization the healthcare manager serves. There are many positions in a medical facility that have management in the title. A few examples are "administrator manager" and "food service manager." The differences come in when you look at the core competencies of healthcare managers. They have to be able to develop plans that can determine the needs of an organization and the direction of a team of medical professionals. They also have to possess the ability to organize management functions within the organization. In addition to this capacity, they will need to be able to work with a staff that will include doctors, nurses, and medical administrative support. Then they have to have an overall ability to control a situation in a professional manner. Finally, they should be able to give directions and make decisions. To do this, they should have conceptual, technical, and interpersonal skills (Thompson, Buchbinder, & Shanks, 2016). A healthcare manager can be found in a variety of roles within a hospital. They get involved with day-to-day staffing concerns, business operations, and

innovative technology that help the hospital provide care for the patients. They will also direct the flow of funds from third party insurers
and others. Their responsibilities can range from helping manage
healthcare teams to ensuring equipment is properly installed. A healthcare manager is in the thick of all hospitals' functions, both internal and
external (Utica, 2016). The issue with all past reform in healthcare is a
primary person was left out the patient care. A healthcare manager is
responsible for the innovation of new technology. They have to understand new reform and teach it to the staff, so they understand the new
standards. They can be responsible for the task that involves patient
care and the daily management of a department within a hospital. A
healthcare manager is responsible for billing and coding in a hospital.
They can also be faced with the need to find free ways to care for a patient, (HBS, 2016). The overall responsibilities of a healthcare manager
would suggest they would be a critical member when it comes to de-
signing a program that could change the way women's health care is
managed.

Other roles that are confused is the clinical manger and healthcare
administration; they seem to be the same job, but they are not. The
two titles are completely different. A healthcare administrative clinical
manager is a supervisor. Many times, they will not get involved directly
with the care of a patient. Their educational requirements are usually
higher also. Most are required to have an MBA. A clinical manager can
get involved with supervising staff and the proper care of a chronically
ill patient. They are responsible for ensuring patient care meets the in-
dustry standards. Their educational requirement can start at a BA
(What is a Clinical Manager in Healthcare Administration, 2016).
Healthcare managers and healthcare administrators operate in slightly
differ ways, but they are also similar. One way is they can both work at
several different types of hospitals at several different levels, depending
on the facility. Healthcare administers can supervise an entire facility.
The major function is to staff the facility with proper employees that

help the service the hospital provides run smoothly. They are also required to have an MBA at the entire level of their job positions (Top Masters in Healthcare, 2016). A clinical manager can work in a single clinic, managing nurses and doctors. They can work directly with patients and staff. They are only required to have a BA at the beginning level of their job. Most have additional clinical education, depending on the field they specialize (What is a Clinical Manager in Healthcare Administration, 2016).

Identifying the Healthcare Professional

The study has identified the differences been between healthcare managers. It has also taken a brief look at the qualitative mandate of the PPACA on other healthcare professionals. So what it looks like is, anyone who is responsible for the health care of a patient can help to develop the needed steps to help women stop suffering in silence and accept that it is okay to speak up when it comes to their health care. The study believes that foundations like the Women's Cancer Fund, which that helps educate, support, and raise funds for the treatment and elimination of cancer, can also help (Women's Cancer Foundation, 2016). Other organizations that can help are the Go Red for Women Association that was established in 2003. Organizations like these are an essential part of the forward solution to help change our society's viewpoint of a woman's role when weighed against her medical needs. The review of the literature suggests that groups like the Go Red for Women and the Cancer Foundation are critical to the change of consciousness necessary to accomplish the change in the morbidity concerns of women in our society. What the literature suggests is any person who is in the position to manage the health care of a patient, whether they are a doctor, nurse practitioner, nurse, or healthcare manager, can help with the phenomenon of silencing the self.

An example could be a doctor who is performing a colonoscopy and has to review a patient's family history. Many things about cancer can be determined from a patient's family history. This doctor may then refer a patient to a genealogy study. In May of 2013, Angelina Jolie took a BRCA 1; this is a test that can determine is a patient has the genes that cause certain cancers. Angelina Jolie did this because her mother, an aunt, and grandmother all died of cancer. She decided that, because the test gave her an 87 percent chance of developing breast cancer and a 50 percent chance of developing ovarian cancer, she would have a double mastectomy (Parry, L, Sep 28, 2015). These types of decisions are the patient's choice. Angelina Jolie can afford to pay for the testing needed to detect the gene that could have caused her cancer. Many women cannot afford the cost of the test. In addition to this factor, if they have health insurance, many doctors will not perform the test because the test is very expensive. The passing of the Affordable Care Act allows free preventive care to women without any cost sharing. The question to ask is, would a test that identifies cancer genes be considered preventive care? Only a medical professional can give an educated answer to this issue. The Affordable Care Act is vital legislation and is crucial to women's health.

Can the New Provisions of the Affordable Care Act Help?

The new provisions of the Affordable Care Act have ensured that women's preventive care is at no cost share for females. It has eliminated the cost-sharing of copay for all preventive care, such as mammograms and screening for cervical cancer (Affordable Care Act Rules on Expanding Access to Preventive Services for Women, 2016). The provision was designed to ensure that by 2013, 73 million individuals would benefit from the preventive care offered by the law (Di Venere,

L., Sep 1, 2012). As of August 2012, the number had reached 47 million. There are eight preventive care services provided under the act. They are well-women visits, gestational diabetes screening, HPV DNA testing, STI counseling, HIV screening and counseling, contraception and contraceptive counseling, breastfeeding support, supplies and counseling, and interpersonal and domestic violence screening and counseling.

The most important part of all these free services is the counseling (Sifferin, A., Aug 1, 2012). The issue is that some women whose economic and social standing is at the low-income level but do not qualify for the Federal Poverty Level standard cannot qualify for the provisions because they cannot afford the cost of health insurance. One reason is they live in states that have not expanded Medicaid, or they are undocumented immigrants. These women cannot afford to pay for insurance on the Marketplace or, in the immigrants' situation, don't qualify for any service due to their citizenship status (Salganicoff, A., Ranji, U., Beamesderfer, A., and Kurani, N., May 15, 2014). So the question here is, how does the healthcare community reach these women in the low-income status who are usually the women that are driving the high levels or morbidity?

Another primary concern is the coverage for abortions. Many women desire an abortion because they cannot afford to take care of another child. It is easy to say just give the child up for adoption, but this act could lead to another psychological issue. Under the Affordable Care Act, abortions are to be paid out of a separate medical fund than the regular healthcare provided. The different collection payment plan puts abortions in a bad light. The provision also gives physicians the right to deny abortions, even if it is due to rape, incest, or the life of the mother is in jeopardy. The difference in the way abortions are treated has become a topic of discussion under the Affordable Care Act (Why the Affordable Care Act Matters for Women: Restriction on Abortion Coverage, Mar 2012). Women are usually the sole parents to children, and the ability to obtain health care for themselves and their children has become a federal concern.

The Affordable Care Act has helped to give more women medical coverage, but we still have a long way to go with achieving this access across all economic and social life situations. If the access to preventive health treatments can help get them connected to the medical professionals that can assist in combating the top 10 morbidity concerns of women's health, how do we get the support for females, no matter the income level? What this shows a missing a crucial part of the issue if the sociological and economic status of women in our society were not examined.

The Affordable Care Act has helped, but what about those cases where women are in poverty and cannot afford the treatment needed to combat the morbidity concerns. Examining the sociological and economic status of women is a very crucial part of the fight against the morbidity concerns of women.

Sociology of Women

Our society is a patriarchy. What this means is males are the dominant force in our community. The have dominion over women and family units. Even though in the last few years women have made considerable changes in education and the workforce, they are still considered unequal to men (Gender Inequality, 2016). The reason for this inequality can be due to the fact women are still paid less than men for the same job. They make less than men by 77.3 percent, and in some states, they make 66 percent less than men (Women & Socioeconomic Status, 2016). The disparity in salaries can account for some of the poverty levels of working mothers in our country. One reason for this could be that even though 38 other countries have been led by women, the United States has never had a woman president (Gender Inequality,

2016). The job of homemaker and mother is fast becoming a second shift after they leave their jobs (Gender Inequality, 2016). This fact is very strange because the amount of women earning higher education has grown at a remarkable rate (The Atlantic, 2016). What makes this fact even stranger is the women in the sociology field have not shown much difference in wages or job positions. The amount of women who function as department chairs in the area of sociology is at the ratio of 40 percent women and 60 percent men. So why is it that it is not the same in those fields that do not require higher education? The inequality between men and women has become acceptable, and no matter the educational level of a woman, the salary or job position is not equal. Women need to be in the positions that will allow them to make decisions about women's issues, like law and social policy, sexual violence, intimidation, harassment, and interpersonal equality (Bailey, M. & DiPrete, T., 2016)

Economics of Women

A woman's economic status is crucial to our country. When a woman can participate on an equal level, it is beneficial to the cities, states, and the nation as a whole (Caiazza, A., Shaw, A. & Werschkul, M., 2016). The reason for this is, when a woman is doing well, her family is also doing well. The better condition of the state of her family will help produce productive citizens. The concern here is leading back to the "silencing the self" phenomenon. We believe we are not good women if we voice our opinions and needs. We also believe that perfection is the only way to prove we deserve what we have worked and earned. Jan Bruce states in her Forbes article that these are restrictive beliefs. In the article, she calls these "beliefs icebergs" (Bruce, J., May 13, 2016). There are six icebergs in our lives. The first is "I lucked into my success." In the end, she says if you are great at your job, you need to own it; no one is that lucky. The next is "the world is not fair." You are right the world is not fair, and getting paid what you earned has nothing to do with being fair but what it is; you are due for a great job (Bruce, J., May 13, 2016). Another is "I need to protect myself from failure." This one is simple: If you never make a mistake, you will never step out to learn new things, and never move forward to achieve bigger and better levels of success. The last three have to do with the perception of people. I have heard the statement perception is truth. Well, if you have the wrong impression, that is your fault, not mine. But women don't think like this way. They believe they have to avoid conflict, make sure people on the job are happy, and they must do everything perfectly. So if you have no conflict, you take no risk and don't get anywhere. Also, you are not responsible for everyone's happiness. The last: No one is perfect. You are from time to time going to make a mistake. Let yourself off the hook, (Bruce, J., May 13, 2016).

Women have to understand how important they are to the economics of our nation. It is estimated that one billion women will be entering our global economy in the next decade. Right now, women are the most underutilized financial asset in the world economy. If the United States, Japan, and Egypt employed women at the same rate as they do men, the GDPs would drop by 5 percent in the United States, 9 percent in Japan, and 34 percent in Egypt (Women and the Economics of Equality, April 2013). The reason for this is because women have chosen to marry at later ages. This change began to occur in 1900. During 1900, only 4 percent of single American women worked (Weigel, M., May 14, 2016). Since this time, the number has climbed. The increase has also led to women having children later in life or without partners. The reason for this could be lower wages earned by men or a lack of job security. Women are becoming more independent. Foundations like the William and Flora Hewlett Foundation are also emerging that work toward building women's economic status on a national level. These organizations work to help women to have a full and fair opportunity to earn a living. The ultimate goal is to ensure women's work is included in labor force participation and economic productivity and to also ensure that, when policies are created, they include gender specific implication of economic policies are understood. Then finally, the agencies are advocates to help women become better informed and educated to influence the policies that effect women's economic status (Women's Economic Empowerment Strategy, Mar 2015).

Many times, when we look at inequality worldwide, we believe that our country is ahead when it comes to these outcomes. The United States has been studying the concerns of women economic status for years. It is true that the recent increase of women who have higher education has improved their social and economic standing, but we still have a long way to go. There are still economic imbalances in women across the lines of race, ethnicity, and region. The continual study of women in these areas will ensure women continue to contribute as full and equal partners in work, politics, and community life. As stated above, when they can do this, it unleashes the potential of the city, state, or nation they live (Women and the Economics of Equality, April 2013).

CDC Report, 10 Leading Causes of Death All Ages, Females, United States 1998-2013

98	99	2000	2001	2002	2003	200
Heart Disease	Heart Disease	Heart Disease	Heart Disease	Heart Disease	Heart Disease	Heart Disease
Malignant Neoplasm	Malignant Neoplasm	Cancer	Cancer	Cancer	Cancer	Cancer
Cardio Disease	Cardio Disease	Stroke	Stroke	Stroke	Stroke	Stroke
COPD	Chronic Lower Respiratory	Chronic Lower Respiratory	Chronic Lower Respiratory	Chronic Lower Respiratory	Chronic Lower Respiratory	Chronic Lower Respira
Pneumonia Flu	Diabetes	Diabetes	Diabetes	Alzheimer's	Alzheimer	Alzheim
Diabetes	Influenza Pneumonia	Influenza Pneumonia	Alzheimer's	Diabetes	Diabetes	Uninten Injuries
Accidents	Accidents	Alzheimer	Unintentional Injuries	Unintentional Injuries	Unintentional Injuries	Diabetes
Alzheimer	Alzheimer	Unintentional Injuries	Influenza Pneumonia	Influenza Pneumonia	Influenza Pneumonia	Influenza Pneumo
Nephritis	Nephritis	Kidney Disease	Kidney Disease	Kidney Disease	Kidney Disease	Kidney Disease
Septicemia	Septicemia	Septicemia	Septicemia	Septicemia	Septicemia	Septicen

	2007	2008	2009	2010	2011	2013
	Heart Disease	Heart Disease	Heart Disease	Heart Disease	Heart Disease	Heart Disease
	Cancer	Cancer	Cancer	Cancer	Cancer	Cancer
	Stroke	Stroke	Stroke	Stroke	Stroke	Chronic Lower Respiratory
tory	Chronic Lower Respiratory	Chronic Lower Respiratory	Chronic Lower Respiratory	Chronic Lower Respiratory	Chronic Lower Respiratory	Stroke
er's	Alzheimer's	Alzheimer's	Alzheimer's	Alzheimer's	Alzheimer's	Alzheimer's
tional	Unintentional Injuries	Unintentional Injuries	Unintentional Injuries	Unintentional Injuries	Unintentional Injuries	Unintentional Injuries
s	Diabetes	Diabetes	Diabetes	Diabetes	Diabetes	Diabetes
a nia	Influenza Pneumonia	Influenza Pneumonia	Influenza Pneumonia	Influenza Pneumonia	Influenza Pneumonia	Influenza Pneumonia
	Kidney Disease	Kidney Disease	Kidney Disease	Kidney Disease	Kidney Disease	Kidney Disease
mia	Septicemia	Septicemia	Septicemia	Septicemia	Septicemia	Septicemia

Color Key for Chart

Heart Disease and Cardiac Illnesses: Yellow is the color for any illnesses that concern cardio-health problems.

Influenza & Pneumonia: Red is for any illnesses that causes difficulty breathing.

Kidney Disease: Orange is for any illnesses that deals with the kidneys.

Septicemia: Turquoise is for any type of infection in the blood stream.

Alzheimer's: Magenta is for any type of brain disorder.

Diabetes: Ocean blue is for illnesses that include high or low blood sugars.

Cancer: Bright green is for any cancers

Conceptual Framework

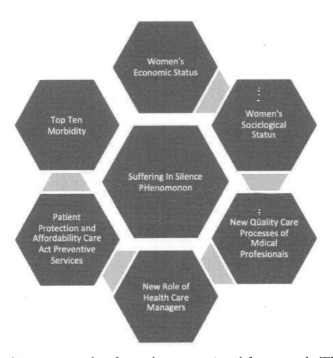

The graph is an example of a study conceptional framework. The middle section is the problem that is being researched. The name is "suffering in silence" common conscious phenomenon that has been described in an article that is identified condition called silencing the self. It referred to the experience of women who suffered from premenstrual syndrome (Perz, J., & Ussher, J. M., Nov 2006). The purpose of the study is to show women silence themselves when it comes to all their medical issues. The study suggested this may be the reason for many of the same morbidity concern for women are the same starting with 1998 (http://www.cdc.gov/nchs/deaths.htm, CDC, NCHS, 1998). CDC reports will be used to support the interests of that some of the same morbidity illness, diseases, and injuries remain. The statement is also backed up by a speech made by Dr. Bustreo from the World Health Organization in 2015 (Bustreo, F. 2015).

The next two on the top help support other possible reasons for the gap. Both the economic status and the sociology of women support the natural consciousness that causes the "silencing the self" description. The literature suggests that women not only use this type of natural knowledge in health but in life. So, when you look at it, the problem is, women will suffer in silence in many other aspects of their lives (Bruce, J., May 13, 2016). They show another woman on the outside but could be unhappy in many other areas of their lives on the inside.

The bottom three blocks refer to the suggested solutions for the problem. The Patient Protection and Affordable Care Act (PPACA) have a portion that is centered on women's health. The no cost sharing for preventive care can help women to get the preventive care that will contribute to identifying the issues in the earlier stages (Sifferlin, A., Aug 1, 2012). The next is to move towards the direction of health management. My research questions surround how healthcare professionals can help manage women's health and who in the medical community would be best to handle the concern. The questions have to include all medical professionals because choosing one would be biased. The PPACA has changed all the role of physicians, nurse practitioners, nurses, and even administrators. It is important to show these recent changes because the PPACA has also changed the way the medical community handles women's services.

Theory of Research Framework

The two theories that have come to the surface of the study are:

Theory 1

Women silence the self because they and society have the same expectation that believe a well put together women is one who is calm, pleasant, and happy all the time. She will always put the needs of her family first and never make waves.

Theory 2

Women believe if they show weakness, they will not achieve the success they are striving to reach. In a man's world, they are lucky to get the advances they have and need to maintain those advances by not making too many waves.

Summary of Literature Review

The phenomenon of silencing the self is real and has become socially acceptable to not just our society, but to women. The definition of the event is when a woman has the outer appearance of a well put together woman who is calm and completely in control of her emotions. She does not make waves or cause any conflict. The truth is, she is a different woman inside. She could be angry, dissatisfied with aspects of her life or job, or even be in pain or discomfort from a medical concern, but no one knows because she will never voice it to anyone (Perz, J., & Ussher, J. M., Nov 2006). Women are still so very important to our nation, but the fact is, cardiovascular disease claims the lives of at least 500,000 American women a year, and this is just too many (About Go Red, 2016). Heart disease and heart-related illness are one, three, and four, and have remained the same for 16 years, but there are still seven more.

We also need to think about the changes in women sexuality. Our healthcare community is not adequately trained to meet the concerns of the lesbian or gay community. Whether we agree with their chosen lifestyles or not, they are entitled to health care. The inability to deal with the health needs of lesbians is just another example of an area of women's healthcare that is overlooked, and the overlooking of the concern is accepted as normal (Helfrich, C. A. & Simpson, E. K., 2006).

Preventive service can become a way for all healthcare professionals to start developing the mindset that would stop the practice of suffering in silence. Healthcare professionals still need to develop the relationships that would foster a better mindset in women. It could help by making women feel more comfortable with talking with their regular practitioners about their concerns. There is also a need for the practitioner to take back control of the health care visit. When a woman goes to the doctor, they know what they want. They are usually on the way to a family function, and going to the physician is more like going through a drive-through and ordering food. They want to be in and out and on with life. Healthcare professionals need to slow them down, take control of the visit, and take care of their health concerns. Helping them to focus on self will help develop the proper management of attention they needed to reduce the morbidity levels we see for women.

Women are wonderful creatures who have been brought up to handle five things at one time. Getting women to focus on their health is going to be hard, but it can be done (Anderson, R. T., Barbara, A., M., Weisman, C., Scholle, S., H., Binko, J., Schneider, T., Freund, K., & Gwinner, V., 2001). The reason for this is not because they don't care, are uneducated about their health, or even that they don't have time. It is because women are the caregivers of the world. Women must not just teach but lead and inspire generations of men and women to be their best. They have to be tough in the world they live. The way they do this is to make the sacrifices it takes to achieve their goals of world caregivers. The only issue is that sacrifice should not have to come at the price of their lives. The people women influence will still need them for years after they embark on their life journey.

The other goal would also be to help change the acceptance of society. It has become natural to accept the phenomena of suffering in silence that has created the same ongoing conditions that have affected women's health since 1998 as reported by the CDC.

Chapter Three

Health care has come a long way when dealing with women's health concerns and issues. There is still a long way to go, but it seems we are circling the same problems. My research examines this from a "suffering in silence" viewpoint. Some women know a lot about their health care and others don't. No matter what economic or ethical race they come from, this rule rings true. Women have a tendency to say, "If it gets worse, I will go to the doctor. Today I have a to-do list that does not have time to go to the physician." Some illnesses have symptoms like bloating and cramping that are not unusual to women's health when taken on an individual basis. When they are put together with others, they may be too busy to acknowledge there could be a serious issue. They suffer in silence because no one wants to deal with a complaining woman. The good wife and mother never complain (Perz, J. & Ussher, J. M., Nov 2006).

The methodology for my research is qualitative. My research will be done in a survey with eight essay questions. Over the last year, my research questions have changed, and my bias and assumptions have been resolved. In the beginning, because I had some personal experiences that colored my thoughts about my research topic, I did not see the gray spaces. When I was able to see the gray areas, I saw the gap in the science. Some articles directly address the suffering of women when it comes to their health care. Still, many others suggest the suffering in silence phenomena. My research will begin to examine the suffering in silence events. Because there is a vast amount of existing material that covers the topic of women's health, it is a well-covered research question. As I stated above, many articles suggest there is a silent side of women's suffering but because the science in them is more about the illnesses, the topic is touched upon very vaguely. My research will bring this out and bring out a possible connection in the science to a new way of combating women's health care concerns and issues.

Research Tradition

The phenomenon of silencing the self was one that was initially studied in 2006. It stated that women who suffer from premenstrual issues do in silence. They accept the idea that a real woman is one who never complains and is always pleasant, no matter what they are experiencing. Women who suffer from premenstrual issues are usually in a large amount of pain. They never share this fact with anyone around them. The phenomenon can also cause women to become depressed and have a poor self-perception. The psychological aspect of the study will not be covered in this study but is an area that needs further research (Perz, J. & Ussher, J. M., 206). The research study theory is that this condition not only affects premenstrual syndrome, but it also expands to all women issues. Silencing the self is not only a subjective consciousness of women, but society. The unspoken expectation is that women get it done no matter the issue. They do everything without complaint and present themselves as calm well put together people who are invincible. Women make sacrifices for society at all levels of life. When you look at the top 10 morbidity concerns starting in 1998, you see the same 10 medical issues. These reports are the basis of the expansion of the silencing the self-phenomenon.

Research Questions and Propositions

The research theory is one that is committed to medical professionals taking responsibility for females to stop suffering in silence and beginning a way forward to change continual concerns of women health since 1998. The research question is the proposed as follows:

> **RQ:** What process can be put into place within the medical community to assist women in receiving quality health care, and how might leaders of these organizations be held accountable?

Many studies have been done on education when it comes to women's health. There have also been many studies on the illnesses and disease that concern women. This research is centered on why in our society there is still high morbidity the same 10 conditions since 1998 (Leading Causes of Death by Age Group, All Females-United States, 1998-2013).

Research Design

The research will be set up with a copy of the CDC reports graph, the list of the eight preventive treatments that are provided by the Patient Protection and Affordability Care Act, and a definition of the phenomenon of "silencing the self." This information will be given to help the participants to understand the study better. The survey will be placed on different medical professionals. The list of professionals will be physicians, nurse practitioners, nurses, and healthcare managers or administrators. The survey will consist of seven open-ended questions that relate to the CDC report, eight preventive care no cost sharing provisions, and the definition of the "silencing the self" phenomenon.

Population and Sample

It would seem my population would be women, but it is not. The community I want to focus on is healthcare professionals. They are the key to the future of the science. The role of the medical professionals has changed due to the Affordable Care Act (Lagace, M., 2016). The law requires a higher quality of care. It also provides free preventive services for women. When women get the scheduled preventive care, it will lead to earlier diagnosis (HHS.gov, 2016). The study leans towards the thought that preventive care is the way ahead in the science of women's health. This is why the provisions of the PPACA are part of the study.

My study is a qualitative study that has been studied several times. The definition of the survey leans towards an intermediate theory research process. There will be careful analysis a survey that will be given to 10 healthcare professionals in the Augusta community (Edmondson, A. C. & McManus, S. E., 2007). My sampling will be made up of doctors, nurse practitioners, nurses, and healthcare managers. The reason for this is the study also has a question which medical professional could provide the best service for female health concerns. The study will be comprised of open-ended questions that lead the experts to give narratives of concerns they have and open communication about the way ahead in the science. The analysis of the study will be done by examining repeat words and phrases found in the responses to the study. Because it is an intermediate study that is designed to look at women's health from a different perspective, accurate evaluation of the survey responses is required (Edmondson, A. C. & McManus, S. E., 2007).

My resource will be an emailed survey to a sampling of medical professionals in the community. Augusta is a medical town, and finding a good mix of professionals should be easy. The researcher chose to use email as the deliverability process to show respect to time management for the medical professionals. This method will also help me to have written data to analyze from each participant.

Sampling Procedure

The sampling procedure is based on the current atmosphere of treatment for women. In most cases, women will be treated by a nurse practitioner. There is also a change in the way healthcare managers and administrators operate since the new Patient Protection and Affordable Care Act (PPACA), so they will also be part of the survey process. Because the question of responsibility is part of the study, other healthcare professionals will be included in the review. The other specialist will be nurses, and of course, you cannot do a medical staff review without including physicians. The sampling size will be a total of 10 participants. The breakdown will be three nurse practitioners, two doctors, three healthcare managers and administrators, and two nurses.

Instrumentation

Many survey instruments can be used on the internet. I am going to use a survey as the tool in this research study. The questions will directly relate to the eight preventive provisions in the Patient Protection and Affordability Care Act, the CDC reports from 1998 to 2013, and the definition of "silencing the self." There will be seven open-ended essay questions.

Validity

There will be a survey used for the research process. With the inquiry a copy of the CDC reports from 1998 to 2013, a list of the eight preventive, no cost sharing treatments provided by the Patient Protection and Affordability Care Act, and the definition of the "silencing the self" phenomenon. The questions in the survey will be deal directly with these three foundational theories of the study.

The last question in the survey will also give the medical professionals the opportunity to give an example of a process they believe will improve women's health care and change the morbidity concerns of women in the United States. By providing the foundational information, it will help to get the present-day professionals' opinions on whether they agree with the study. It will also give them an opportunity to deliver an opinion of the present-day concerns of women's health. The continuing process of collecting data from the medical professionals who work in the field will also give a further research perspective for the study. By providing these three findings of the research associated with this study, it will give the participants information needed to give dependability, creditability, and confirmation to the study (Creswell, J. W., 2014). The combined analysis of the CDC reports and the definition of the "silencing the self" phenomenon (Perz, J. & Ussher, J. M., Nov 2006) coupled with the list of eight no cost-sharing provisions and survey results will help to triangulate the study and give it validity(Creswell, J. W., 2014).

Reliability

[For reliability, the researcher must ascertain whether the instrument(s) consistently gather(s) the same information over time and circumstance.

There's an assumption that accompanies this; what is being measured stays the same over time. As you can imagine, this may be difficult to ascertain in some studies. However, when (esp.) quantitative instruments are employed, the researcher must provide evidence of the reliability of the device. It is likely that you use Test-Retest Reliability measures and Inter-rater reliability measures.]

Data Collection

Augusta is a medical town, and women's health has become a primary focus in the city. An example of this is the recent opening of a women's health care clinic in the VA Hospital in Augusta, GA. Many of the medical professionals in the Augusta area are willing to participate in the survey. There are also clinics in other medical facilities that are working on projects like the one I am doing and would be great resources to find other medical professionals who would like to participate in the study.

While I am only looking for 10 responses, I will give out additional surveys. The process of delivering these surveys will be by electronic mail. I chose this delivery process because medical professionals are very busy, and this will give them the opportunity to do the questionnaire in at their leisure. The thought process behind this is they can type in the answers and have more time to give thought to their answers. The survey will be returned to me by email with a return time of no more than 30 days. If I have not received at least 10 reviews back in 30 days, I do a follow-up email with a read response attached. This will allow me to track the response to my survey and know who is actively reading the emails.

While the emails will identify the professionals by name, once the surveys are downloaded to my computer, there will be no names attached to them. Once I receive three reviews from three nurse practitioners, two physicians, three healthcare managers and administrators, and two nurses, I will send out thank you response to all participants whether they filled out the survey or not.

Data Analysis

An exploratory qualitative methodology was selected over other qualitative designs because the focus of the research was to categorize and interpret themes (Creswell, 2014). Qualitative data analysis methods were conceptual and relational (Writing@CSU: Writing Guide, 2016). Conceptual data analysis involved establishing the presence of themes. Relational data analysis begins with the identification of present concepts and continues by looking for semantic relationships (Writing@CSU: Writing Guide, 2016). Semantic relationships were established using thematic units. Thematic units were high-level abstractions interpreted from underlying themes and patterns built in the qualitative data (Linguistics, 201, 2016). Data analysis process involved the emergence of topics from the interview transcripts and other collected data, such as the personal journal.

Data analysis begins by organizing the collected information followed by data perusal, classification, and synthesis (Elo, Kaariainen, Kanste, Polkki, Utrianinen, & Kyngas, 2014). The data analysis approach for exploratory analysis includes (a) compiling the data from the interviews, (b) organizing the data by interviewee, (c) coding of the data (i.e., organizing the data by recognized categories), (d) identifying themes (i.e., the label attached to each designated group), and (e) establishing data relationships (i.e., recognizing similarities and differences in themes in order to condense or separate themed categories, as appropriate) (Saunders, Lewis, & Thornhill, 2012). Once this process is completed, the established themed classes are the findings of the study.

The coding rules that would be used to map textual units into data terms included developing the aspects of interpretation to formulate the material into categories that represent the theme of the study (Mayring, 2009). The technique that would be used to translate data terms into themes is inductive category development (Mayring, 2009).

The topics and combinations of issues would be recorded by analyzing the similarities of the participants to the objective of the research question (Mayring, 2009).

A deductive analysis tool would be used to determine the similarities of the participant's responses to the research question (Mayring, 2009). The deductive analysis tool provided ability to research with the capacity to determine similarities between the participant's responses. It also helped to identify a theme that relates to the research question, (Mayring, 2009).

Ethical Considerations

The ethical principles applied throughout the research process would involve informing the participants of the right to have a safe environment for the interview. It also included receiving an informed consent form (see Appendix C) and explaining a participant's right to terminate the interview without giving a reason for ending the interview (Rubin & Rubin, 2012). Each interviewee would sign an informed consent form before his or her interview begins. The participant's identity would be protected by assigning numbers to the interview transcripts. The only person who would know the identity of the number and participant is the researcher. All data that was collected would be on the researcher's password protected email, computer, and iPhone.

To ensure the highest level of ethical research, principles of the Belmont Report protocol would be maintained. The Belmont Report principles primarily focus on the well-being of study subjects (Bromley,

Mikesell, Jones, & Khodyakov, 2015). The vulnerable research population must be protected from potential exploitation (Rogers & Lange, 2013). In this study there were no vulnerable participants. Also, the three principles of the Belmont Report protocol (i.e., autonomy, beneficence, and justice) would be maintained (Strause, 2013). In this study the participant's identities would be protected by assigning each interview a number. The researcher would be the only person who had access to the information. The information would be stored on a password protected personal computer that was used for the researcher's academic studies. The researcher does not allow the computer to be used by anyone else.

Researchers must ensure no harm comes to participants due to participation in a study (Rubin & Rubin, 2014). Risks must also be minimized to participants. To ensure awareness of the risks and benefits of the proposed study, each participant would be required to sign an informed consent form (see Appendix C). The consent form includes (a) the purpose of the study, (b) the involvement of participates, (c) participation procedures, (d) the benefits of the research, (e) the risks of taking part, (f) costs and compensation, (g) confidentiality, (h) voluntary nature of participating, and (i) the rights of the participant to withdraw (Wright, 2012).

Biases could occur due to preexisting knowledge and experience with the topic (Creswell, 2014). Bias would be mitigated by using open-ended questions during the interview, focusing solely on the responses of participants, performing triangulation, and using note taking. Another way the investigated worked to eliminate bias was to interview both men and women. The purpose was to eliminate the natural bias of the females. The investigator has experienced that females, no matter their profession or career level, have a horror story about the medical care they or someone close to them had received. The conflict of interest to the researcher was the loss of three key women in the researcher's life. The researcher would use a journal to ensure any personal feelings or concerns are recorded during the interview process. The process of writing down the researcher's personal feelings would help to identify potential conflicts related to the researcher's personal bias.

Summary of Chapter Three

Exploratory qualitative research provided the researcher with a process that provided similar responses from participants to help answer the study research question. An exploratory qualitative approach was best because the study would use an interview to collect data (Creswell, 2014).

Data would be gathered from ten participants. These participants would be from the Southeast regions of the United States. Purpose sampling would be used. Semi-structured interview questions would be utilized. Data analysis would follow the general approach described by inductive analysis (Mayring, 2009). The information in the study was designed to provide data that would contribute to the development of relevant parameters of a medical guideline for improving the quality of women's health care.

Chapter Four

Chapter Four presents a collection of data that supported the explorative qualitative approach of the study. Chapter Four provides analysis of the research study that surrounds relevant guidelines that can improve the quality of women's health care. Women's health came to the forefront of consciousness in the 1970s (Salganicoff, 2013). Since that time women's mortality and morbidity rates have been as high as 42.7 percent in the United States (Nisen, 2014). The purpose of the exploratory qualitative study was to discover the relevant parameters of a medical guideline for improving the quality of women's health care. The overarching research question is, "what are the relevant parameters for a medical guideline for improving the quality of women's health care?" The chapter contains the demographics of the participants of the study and the data collected from one-on-one interviews. The interviews were conducted in-person using a semi-structured interview style. The investigator allowed the participants to speak freely and used probing questions to ensure a complete and definite understanding of the participants' responses. The research process used an inductive approach to identify similarities in the participants' responses. The study was designed to allow health care administrators to give their honest opinions on how they feel about being included in the initial decisions concerning the quality of care for women's health. The content of this chapter involves the explanation of the data analysis and information that gives a clear description of the interviews. Chapter four includes the participant demographics, the presentation of the data collected, and a summary of the findings of the exploratory qualitative study.

Participant Demographics

The participants in the study were retired health care administrators that lived in the Southeast. They worked in the health care administrative areas for at least ten years. Most of them had more than 20 years of experience, and they still had regular activity in a medical facility. They all showed a deep concern for the health care system and its success. They also demonstrated a sincere desire to help patients to achieve the best medical care and with positive outcomes to their health situations. They also had work experience in both a clinical and hospital setting. There were four male participants and six female participants. The reason for interviews with male medical professionals was to get their thoughts on how well they felt female patients were cared for in the health care system. Having male participants also helped to give another viewpoint about women's health care. The purpose was to eliminate the natural bias of the females. The investigator has experienced that women, no matter their profession or career level, have a horror story about the medical care they or someone close to them had received.

All participants were sent consent forms to the emails they provided to the investigator. No interviews were conducted before a consent form was signed by the participant. Each interview was uploaded into Rev.com. The application transcribed the audio recording of the interview into a Word Document. Once the copied documents were returned, the participants were sent a copy of the Word Document so they could verify their responses before the data was included in Chapter Four. The table below illustrates participant demographics (see Table 1). Each participant met the criteria for the study that were set by the investigator. The criteria were that each participant had to be a retired patient administrator. They had to have at least ten years of experience as a patient administrator. They also had to have worked in both a hospital and a clinical setting. Then finally they had to be located in the Southeastern Region of the United States.

Table 1

Participant Demographics

Participant	Gender	Years of Experience
P1	Male	25
P2	Male	22
P3	Female	21
P4	Female	15
P5	Male	20
P6	Female	18
P7	Male	20
P8	Female	20
P9	Female	23
P10	Female	21

Presentation of the Data

Interviews that were conducted used semi-structured questions to collect data. The investigator also used probing questions to ensure clarification of the participants' responses (see Appendix C). The literature presented in Chapter 2 of this paper showed that women's health care in the United States needs work. The issue was not that research had not been done. It was determined that the findings of past research be valid. The issue is that there was an inconsistency of translating the data that was collected into the laws that would develop guidelines that could be used by doctors to treat female patients (IOM, 2010).

This process was also supported by the research by pointing out that the new Patient Protection and Affordable Care Act made a particular focus on women's health care (Sebelius, 2011). This section presents representative and aggregated data from the ten participants who responded to the interview questions found in Appendix B. Data was coded to identify major themes that represent the findings of this study. The investigator utilized an inductive method to determine the similarities in the participants' responses.

Question One Data

Question one asked, "What are medical guideline parameters the most successful in improving women's health care?" The themes for question one were preventive care and education. Under prevention, the secondary findings were self-check and self-examinations that start with the patient and annual, periodical, and different medical screening connected to the patient's medical and family history that should be done on a regular basis. These are referenced as the most important things that are done to support the success of women's health care. The next theme was the education for both patients and medical professionals. The need to educate women about their bodies is one of the subthemes that appeared when it came to the success of women's health. The other subtheme under education was that physician's need better understanding and teaching on the conditions that would require them to refer their female patients to specialty care.

Other secondary themes were the part males play both when developing policies and procedures concerning women's health. Also, their perceptions of the need for additional funding when it comes to developing programs relating to women's health was a concern by participants. Some other concerns were the level of communication and listening skills of male physicians. This was mentioned by two male participants and only one female participant. The overarching themes in response to question one were that preventive health exams and educational programs relating to women's health were done well. P2 made this point by stating "the only parameters that I can think of that are most successful is education." P5 also made this point by saying "annual and periodical physicals drastically help the awareness and immediate intervention to prevent health issue that can escalate and veer out of control." All of the participants made mention of education, and the eight out of ten of them suggested preventive care.

Question Two Data

Question two asked, "What medical parameters are used for all patients?" The themes for question two were also education and prevention. These two themes intersected with each other. The subthemes included early intervention at childhood with teaching children to eat well, exercise, and develop healthy habits. The thought pattern of the participant was that children would grow up to be healthier adults that were more involved in staying healthy and doing those things to take care of themselves. Other subthemes emerged about teaching adults to take control of habits that will cause problems with their health or decrease the quality of their life and longevity. P7 made this point by stating, "Lifestyle is important, make sure if they are smoking or drinking or something, and just make sure that either not to smoke, or not to drink, or to limit what they do in their control." P1 made this point by stating, "All patients are education. In today's society, of course, all health care is going to preventive." The overall educational theme was developing programs to teach patients through the process of outreach programs. These programs would include preventive care, by teaching healthy life habits to children.

Additional subthemes surfaced about male dominance that concerned their control over the decisions that affected the policies and procedures that governed women's health care and how it is conducted. P2 made this point by stating, "That is specific clinics for women, but overall, the care is male-driven". P10 made this point by saying, "I think the male gets more care through the specialty than the female". The other secondary subtheme was the importance of women being referred to specialty care like a cardiovascular referral, women's specialty clinics, and pediatric hospitals.

Notable points were the consistent and persistent responses about starting early with children to develop healthy life habits that will affect their overall quality of life and health. The suggestions for continuing in the process of reaching children at an earlier age were to develop community outreach programs that deal with social and economic issues that will lead to better health care decisions. P8 made this point by stating, "There are more parameters for all patients than there are for women and I think that we can look at what we do for children."

Question Three Data

Question three asked, "Which of these guidelines for all patients are the most important?" The themes for question three were education and community outreach. The themes for this issue interlocked like the themes in questions two and three. The theme of teaching was important because it focused on the need for developing programs that started at a young age. The outreach programs could be used to establish processes that teach healthy eating and exercising habits. They would also be used to develop better social and economic environments that could support the development of relevant parameters in health care that could improve women's quality of life in the United States. P7 made this point by stating, "what's most important is the lifestyle, what are you doing, what are you eating, how are you taking care of yourself, your rest and your exercising." These themes intersected with community outreach. They could be used to accomplish higher educational goals for patients and health care providers. The majority of participants mentioned the need to increase community outreach where children and families lived.

The subthemes of preventive health care and doctor-patient relationships surround the need for more awareness about what is going on in the communities that surround the hospital and clinics. Community outreach, preventive care, education, and the patient-doctor relationship could help improve the health care of that patient who did not get the regular care he or she needed. While training and community outreach are necessary, if the patient does not have adequate access to care with a medical provider, the lack of access could cause additional hindrance in improving the health. P2 made this point by stating, "I would say definitely ... For me, I think the most important would be access to care, preventive education." P6 made this point by stating, "Just get them to the door. We have first to figure out why they are not coming". The striking statement was the medical community needs to be proactive in finding out why patients are not getting the preventive care they need. Is it because individuals do not have the money, need to pay bills instead, or maybe they have no transportation? The overall interlocking theme in question three was that outreach services would help develop relevant parameter guidelines that would improve the quality of care for all patients', not just women.

Question Four Data

Question four asked, "Which of these guidelines for all patients are the least important?" The theme for question four was that all the participants agreed that there was not a guideline that was least important. P3 made this point by stating, "I would not say that there's a least important. I think they are all just as important because when it comes to saving a life, I think all things should be considered." They did mention concerns about ways to develop better deliverance of quality health care. Most of the participants still stressed the need for both better outreach and education. They also continued to state the need to reach children at an early age. Getting outreach programs set up in rural communities and creating outreach programs that focused on the elderly were some of the suggestions. P2 made this point by stating, "In this country that we have the worst outreach programs when it comes to bringing people into the health care system." There was mention of the natural practices of not paying any attention to one's health until he or she is in his or her 30s, 40s, and 50s, which was considered to be too late. The health care community should be taking a more proactive stance when it comes to patients with this mindset. P1 made this point by stating, "Folks think that because they do not have issues, then they do not need to go in." The development of a better doctor-patient relationship and addressing patient concerns was another method that was mentioned that could improve the effectiveness of outreach programs. The emphasis on outreach programs leads back to the importance of developing relevant parameters that would improve the quality of health care for all patients.

Question Five Data

Question five asked, "How will these guidelines for all patients improve women's health care?" The themes for question five were education, the doctor-patient relationship, and outreach programs. The responses made by the participants under education were centered on teaching people how to live better and make healthier life choices. The subtheme under education concerning early intervention at early primary school level was also connected to teaching women how to stay healthy. Use of wellness clinics was a suggestion for increasing the effectiveness of preventive health care programs that encouraged wellness. P7 made this point by stating, The prevention measure starts when they're young, and I was saying pediatrics, if we had more pediatrics wellness clinics that mothers, after they have their children, they could teach their children how to eat, how to be whole, instead of letting our kids eat all this stuff.

If the health care community could develop wellness programs for women and families, five of the participants stated that this would lead to quality lives and quality health. Seven out of ten participants noted that healthy habits lead to healthy minds, bodies, souls, and behaviors.

The overall theme stated by all participants was that of teaching women to develop habits that encourage proper diet, rest, and exercise. The thought process was that development of guidelines that focused on these teachings would lead to healthy young girls with good habits. These young girls would grow up to have healthy babies, and the quality of life would become a generational practice.

The second theme was doctor-patient relationships. This theme could lead to better health care because it could develop the type of open relationships that would help women be more comfortable and open with their physicians. Illness does exist, and when women feel comfortable, they are more likely to share their concerns. When doctors know the family health history of their patients, they can use this information to treat their female patients more effectively. Lastly, the mention of having more female doctors could contribute to improving the quality of health care available for women.

Another secondary theme was about outreach. Responses focused on developing a program that works with education to teach wellness and develop other programs to assist the family in developing healthy life habits. Teaching mothers how to care for their family and reaching young girls in their natural environments was also a process that could help families develop healthy living habits. Using education as a theme to improve preventive care was stressed. Finally, the process of teaching patients how to develop relationships with physicians that encourage open communication could help the medical community to develop outreach programs with educational themes that could lead to wellness in women's health care.

Question Six Data

Question six asked, "What improvements are needed for all patient parameters?" The themes that emerged for question six intertwined with each other. They were education, barriers to health care and improvement in the delivery of health care by doctors. The improvements identified were developing programs that would encourage better habits and improve their patient's quality of life. The way ahead was reaching children in the communities where they live and the schools they attend. Also if medical professionals work with outreach programs that educate mothers to help feed their families better meals, it would improve the quality of health for these individuals. In addition to educating patients, it was suggested that medical professionals need help developing better relationships with patients. The education would include retraining for those doctors who have been in practice for many years that did not know how to communicate with the patient. Empathy training could also help to develop skills that would show more concern for patients and their quality of life. P1 made this point by stating, "educating our staff members, teaching them how to present themselves to our patient." P1 also made this point by saying, "it starts with the providers, it starts with that staff member, it starts with the customer service that we provide to our women out there."

It was also suggested that there was a need to develop systems that help with better access to care. This process could be done by addressing language barriers and looking into better access to insurance for the patient who could not afford insurance. Developing a better system in the United States that focused on more patients being able to access the care they need at a price they could afford was emphasized. P2 made this point by stating, "One barrier to everyone when it comes to health care is cost and the obstacles that we have created to access to care." The most concerning point is that the health care system is built on treating the patient who is already sick. It is a process that depends on people being sick to make money. The system seems to prey on the ill and does not teach patients how to stay healthy. P8 made this point by stating, "It is just so sad that our whole business is about money and people being sick. It is kind of like we prey on that." The rising cost of health care could decrease if there were policy changes that assisted medical professionals to be more proactive in catching illnesses before it is too late. P7 made this point by stating, "The health care community, of course, needs to be more proactive in getting folks involved in a lot of different activities." The process of teaching wellness, not sickness and meeting people in their communities was considered instrumental to most of the participants in developing the relevant parameter guidelines to improve the quality of health care. P8 made this point by stating, "We need preventive measures and find parameters to make people well. It all goes back to wellness. Why couldn't we be a wellness hospital, instead of a hospital where everybody is sick?"

Question Seven Data

Question seven asked, "What specific medical guideline parameters should be improved for women's health?" The theme for question seven is responsibilities. The responsibilities of doctors to patients enhance their relationships with their patients. It was also mentioned that it is the patient's responsibilities to follow the instructions from their doctors. When it comes to medical treatment physicians, do have a certain amount of responsibility. However, a patient also has some responsibilities. P1 made this point by stating, "It got to be an open relationship, it got to be a committed relationship, and both parties got to be dedicated." The theme that there needed to be an environment that supported a system of patient-centered health care that developed healthy habits to create wellness. P1 made this point by stating, "It is patient-centered care now that is what we are going into is patient-centered care. The patient is the driver. The patient determines which direction he or she wants to go". The other concern that was noted was the growing mental health issues of women. Female patients needed to be more proactive when dealing with stressors in their lives. They needed to put their health first and develop healthy mindsets that foster mental and emotional balance in their lives and their families' lives. P6 made this point by stating, I think if we can get that psychological and that emotional treatment that women need to be able to deal or to delegate or to get some help with what's stressing them out, with what is too overbearing, with what is too much for them. I think the health stuff will fall in line.

It was also suggested that health care professionals need to learn more about developing relationships with patients. They also need to develop programs that will help them to meet their patients in their environment. In addition to meeting patients in their surroundings, health care professionals need to be more proactive with patient-centered care, where the patient is an active part of the health care team. This process could develop relationships and build a society of wellness. These guidelines could help women by giving them a safe environment to become mentally, emotionally, and physically healthier. The overall theme was the process of helping females to develop quality mental, emotional, and physical health for themselves and their families to create a practice of wellness that could follow them into adulthood and the communities they live. Developing a system of wellness may contribute to improving the relevant parameters that would create quality care for women's health in the United States.

Question Eight Data

Question eight asked, "What possible issues do you see with developing parameters relevant guidelines to improve women's health?" The theme for question eight was laws. Under laws, there were subthemes about male driven decisions and male doctors who lack understanding for females' specialty needs. P2 made this point by stating, "Congress health care decisions are male-driven when it comes to women's health care." The other subtheme was in regard to the perceptions that people believed that male doctors are better. Other concerns that were mentioned under the theme of law, was state and federal legislation. It was also said that some laws determined how much money the country invested in health care and the process would affect the quality for women. P1 made this point by stating,

> *Deciding what type of classes to give, what kind of health care decisions, what women need for health care, although, it is*

not a panel of women in their along with, of course, with some men, but when it comes to women's health care, if it's not dominated by women health care providers.

An additional subtheme is patient-centered care. The patient can drive some of the quality of her care, but the development of more programs that can help a physician be more proactive when treating patients is a key factor. The programs could also allow the doctor to choose how much time he or she will spend with patients who need more assistance. P1 made this point by stating, "We cannot let future laws or established laws take the determination out of the patient's hands. The patient got to be the one that is the driving tool."

In addition to all of these points, it is also important to include the hospital administrator in the process of health care because he or she drives the flow of patients in the hospital and the funding of procedures and operation of a medical facility. P2 made this point by stating, "The health care administrator is all focused on the money. Driving the hospital, pay for the procedures, paying for that equipment that is the health care administrator." Having all the levels of professionals at the table would help to change the direction of unnecessary spending in the health care system. Once the funds are spent on the correct procedures, the quality of health care should improve. P2 made this point by stating,

> *Financially, because every health care facility is a business first. If they are losing money, then that procedure is going to get cut, but if that health care provider (Administrator) was there at the time that these decisions were made, they could make a more rational or more logical decision.*

The other main concern, when it comes to the laws around women's health care, is the lack of women at the decision-making meetings when it comes to decision making concerning female health care. Women being more proactive in their health care and the decisions that involve their health care could help to make a change in the quality of their care. P2 made this point by stating, "The only way it is going to improve is to include women in the decision."

Question Nine Data

Question nine asked, "What do you think the future parameter guidelines for women's health care should be?" The theme for question nine was centered on women. It dealt with the need for females to be more proactive about all parts of their health care. They need to ensure they get all their preventive care, periodical physicals, and annual exams completed on time. P1 made this point by stating, "To me, preventive care is the only way to improve health care for anybody, not just specifically women." P1 also made this point by stating, "without preventive health care, I think this country right here, would be bankrupt health care-wise." The theme also focused on how women need to be more involved with the laws that concern their health care. Females also need to be more involved in the statues that develop the laws concerning their health care. They also need to be more proactive when making quality of life decisions. The importance is in putting their self and their health first. This subtheme is important because women are the caretakers of the world. Another subtheme that was mentioned addressed the amount of money that is spent in the health care system and how much of it is allocated to women. P1 made this point by stating, "We need more investment, more allocations for women-specific health care."

Question Ten Data

Question ten asked, "In your opinion, what are the current parameters medical guidelines for women's health?" The theme for question ten is that the parameters that surround women's health are actively moving towards better relationships with their physicians and developing a more proactive attitude in women towards their health care. Other factors were that more technology was being used when it comes to women's health. All the participants emphatically noted the concern for health care to be delivered in a more compassionate, empathetic way, with a commitment to physicians and patients. P1 made this point by stating, "Maya Angelou has a famous quote. She says, People would never remember what you said or what you did, but they will remember how you made them feel." There is also growing recognition due to the Affordable Care Act for more women's centered health programs that help with the economic responsibilities. P4 made this point by stating, "It (Affordable Care Act) is almost non-existent as the Government throws women health issues into legislation packaged with the Affordable Care Act to which the current governing body is trying to repeal desperately." The cost of health care can be high but laws that can contribute to women receiving the preventive care that could be used to detect possible issues before they become seriously ill is crucial to developing the parameter guidelines that will improve the amount of attention needed to improve women's health care.

Presentation and Discussion of Findings

The exploratory qualitative research provided the researcher with a data collection process that provided similar responses from participants to help answer the study research question. The data analysis approach for exploratory analysis included (a) compiling the data from the interviews, (b) organizing the data by interviewee, (c) coding data that is structured by recognized categories), (d) identifying themes that attached labels to each designated group, and (e) establishing data relationships that recognized similarities and differences in themes. Then the date was condensed or separated by themes into appropriate categories (Saunders, Lewis, & Thornhill, 2012). Once this process was completed, the established themed classes were then considered the findings of the study.

Data was gathered from ten participants. The participants were interviewed using semi-structured interviews. The study was designed to provide data that would contribute to the development of relevant parameters of a medical guideline for improving the quality of women's health care. From this analysis, four major themes and seven subthemes emerged. These themes are presented below.

Major Themes of the Study

During the interview process, there were four major themes that emerged. These themes were preventive care, education, outreach programs, and physicians' responsibility. Table 2 below shows the themes and the frequency of the themes. The same participants may have mentioned a theme more than once. The table shows how many participants discussed the theme, not how many times a theme was mentioned. What was stated by the majority of participants was that the four major themes were being done well, but they all needed to be done better.

The four major themes provide applicable information to the central research question, which was "what is the relevant parameter for a medical guideline for improving the quality of women's health care?" The four major themes of preventative care, education, outreach, and physician's responsibility draw attention to the needs of patients and improving the quality of care for women in the United States. The participants stated that in the United States that the two major themes were showing improvement included preventive care and education.

Table 2

Frequency of Major Themes

Themes	Frequency
Preventative Care	9 of 10
Education	8 of 10
Outreach	7 of 10
Physician's Responsibility	6 of 10

Major Theme One

Preventive health care was the number one major theme that came from the study. Preventive health care was being done correctly, but there were still some areas that need improvement. How this theme lined up with the purpose of the study, which was to discover the relevant parameters of a medical guideline for improving the quality of women's health care, was that it pointed out areas where preventive health care could be enhanced. The issue that arose from preventive treatment was access to care. Access to care included the issues with affordable care, barriers to care like language, laws that blocked or limited the financing of patient care, and lack of insurance. Preventive care topics also included the lack of responsibilities to patients doctors showed, and the absence of responsibility patients showed to following their physician's instructions. When looking at the subthemes of the study doctor/patient relationship, barriers to health care, quality, specialty care, and quality can all be used to improve preventive health care. Better doctor/patient relationships could improve the quality of health care because these relationships could lead to better understanding between patients and physicians. When women feel comfortable, they are more likely to be more open in their communication with their doctors. Better communication would decrease the language barriers that could cause problems with access to care. Other barriers could be laws that are decided by men concerning women's health care. Also, issues with affordable care and access to health insurance could also cause access to care limitations.

Major Theme Two

Education is the next major theme of the study. The study supported education for both health care professionals and patients. Education was discussed, with a need to start early. The responses also included educating women on how to take care of their families better. An area that the theme of education interlocked with was specialty care. The issue with specialty care is that physicians need better training when it comes to identifying the need for specialty care with their female patients. While education was an area that was considered to be heading in the right direction, there could still be more improvement. The patient needs to ensure she carries out her part of the educational process by being committed to her health care. The patient needs to foster the development of better relationships with her physicians by following the instructions that are given by her doctors. This point would help to answer the overarching research question by focusing on educating women and their medical providers on how to build better communication and improving the quality of women's health care. The participants noted that health care administrators and other medical professionals also have a responsibility to help physicians ensure health care resources are used to develop programs that will keep the major themes of preventive care and education working well in the United States.

Major Theme Three

Outreach programs were the third major theme. The participants identified a problem in that the use and implementation of outreach programs are not being done well. More outreach is needed to help develop better educational programs and preventive care practices that could develop into wellness practices. The programs could decrease health care spending. They could help the medical community to focus on better access to care for all patients. Outreach programs could also generate data for better usage of funds when decisions are made concerning women's health care and how it was conducted. The issue is that the medical community needs to work harder at outreach. Meeting patients in their living environments by starting at schools and the communities around the health care facility would assist in discovering the relevant parameters to improve women's health care. Outreach programs interlocked with all the major themes and the subthemes. The other major themes were preventive health care, education, and physician's responsibility. The major themes related to the area of medical communities responsibilities to reach out and meet their patients in the natural environments. This practice could help them teach diet, exercise, and wellness. The medical community could also find out why patients were not able to get the preventive care they needed. Practitioners could also develop an attitude of responsibility in their patients. Outreach programs could help by developing programs that could foster a mindset that encouraged women to be proactive about their medical care. They could also contribute to promoting wellness in women and their families.

Major Theme Four

Physicians' responsibility is the fourth major theme. The theme centered on what physicians could do to make the delivery of health care better. The major focus was the provision of health care. The theme intertwined with preventive care, education, and outreach programs. Care needs to be delivered in a compassionate and empathic way. There needed to be a buy-in by both patients and doctors. Both the patient and the doctor need to be committed to the relationship. Physicians have a responsibility and a desire to ensure the needs of their patients are met. Some of the issues with directives that concerned time limitations for patient visits could be structured to allow the physician to determine the amount of time they needed to take care of their patients. Doctor's hands could be tied if they are not authorized to determine how much time patients need to treat their patients. Other issues could be the lack of female doctors and women's clinics. The need for women physicians and females' clinic could cause barriers in communication and the process of referring female patients to specialty care they require.

Final Analysis of the Study Themes

Subthemes of the Study

The subthemes shown in Table 3 below all supported the four major themes. The subthemes supported the major themes by emphasizing what is needed to help support the improvement of the quality of health care, specifically, women's health care. These subthemes were doctor/patient relationship, male participation, specialty care, laws, and barriers to health care, quality, and technology health care.

The first subtheme was doctor/patient relationship. Doctor/patient relationship related to all the major themes. Physicians and patients need to work together as a team. Preventive care, education, outreach programs, and physician responsibilities cannot be improved unless doctors and patients work together as a team.

The subthemes of male participation, laws, and barrier to health care intertwine with each other. The continued issues of legislation that govern health care concerning women being primarily decided by males can create a barrier to for improving the quality of health for females. While only four out of ten participants mentioned the subtheme of male dominance in women's health care, it was clear that lack of female input in women's health care could cause a barrier to health care by limiting access to care.

Barriers to health care were also noted as a subtheme of the study. Male dominance in law making when it came to women's health was a concern because of the perceived lack of understanding by males when it came to health care decisions that affect women. One area that showed this was the lack of financing and insurance coverage for specialty care. Women need special attention, the cost of specialty care may not be covered by insurers, and the cost of the care may be high. Both of the subthemes of barriers to health care and the male participation could cause issues when developing processes that could improve the quality of health care for women.

A physician's inability to develop a productive relationship with his or her patient could lead to a doctor not referring a female patient to receive the specialty care needed. The laws that would govern the funds to pay for the specialty care or to increase the time spent with patients by physicians could also cause decreased quality of care. They could also hinder the funding needed for the technical services to provide the specialty care needed by the patient. While the use of technology has increased in health care, the financing of that technology is not always provided. The position in the hospital that has the last word concerning the funding of care is the health care administrator. The health care administrator helps to translate the state and federal laws that govern the operations in a medical facility.

Only one participant spoke about patient-centered health care. Even though there was only one participant that talked about the topic, it connected with the major theme of preventive care, education, and physician responsibilities. The subtheme made a point about preventive care being important because patients need to be reminded that even if they are free of medical issues they stilled need to get regular preventive care treatments. The follow-ups, lab test, and well checks by their physicians could save their lives. Letting the patient make the final decision about her treatment was a key factor when expressing the need for better doctor/patient relationships.

Table 3

Frequencies of Subthemes

Themes	Frequency
Doctor/Patient Relationship	5 of 10
Male Participation	4 of 10
Specialty Care	4 of 10
Laws	3 of 10
Barriers to health care	2 of 10
Quality	2 of 10
Technology	2 of 10

The overarching reach question of, "what are the relevant parameters for a medical guideline for improving the quality of women's health care?" tied into all the major themes and subthemes because they could all be used to enhance the quality of health care for women's health. The four major themes of preventive care, education, outreach programs, and physicians' responsibility, emphasized the accessible content of guidelines that should be developed. The sub-themes of doctor/patient relationship, male participation, specialty care, laws, and barriers to health care, quality, technology, and patient-centered health care reinforce the major themes by giving more detailed areas of directions to help develop the processes to improve the quality of women's health care.

Summary of Chapter Four

Included in Chapter four were study outcomes, findings, data analysis, themes, and subthemes that relate to the problem of the lack of relevant parameters of medical guidelines for improving the quality of women's health care. The investigator used the full data from the participant interviews to present the results of this study. There were ten participants in the study. They were retired health care administrators that had ten years or more of experience in the administrative field. They also lived in the Southeast. There were six women and four men. The reason for including men in the study was to help eliminate the natural bias of women concerning their health care. The use of semi-structured helped the investigator to collect the data that supported the overarching research question, "what are the relevant parameters for a medical guideline for improving the quality of women's health care?" The major themes of the collected data were preventive care, education, outreach programs, and physicians' responsibility. Preventive care and education are being done well, per the views of the study participants, but these areas still need to be improved upon. The majority of the participants believed that preventive care was a major theme when it came to women's health. In addition, there were seven subthemes that emerged from the collected data. The subthemes included doctor/patient relationship, male participation, specialty care, laws, and barriers to health care, quality, and technology.

Chapter Five, the final chapter in this dissertation, pulls the study together by further analyzing the study findings. Chapter Five includes analysis of the gap in the body of knowledge that relates to the purpose of the exploratory qualitative study, to discover the relevant parameters of a medical guideline for improving the quality of women's health care. Chapter Five includes the findings and conclusions, implications, and recommendations for further study of parameter guidelines that would improve the quality of women's health care in the United States. Final conclusions for the dissertation are made at the end of Chapter Five.

CHAPTER FIVE

The purpose of the exploratory qualitative study was to discover the relevant parameters of a medical guideline for improving the quality of women's health care. The issues that were identified in Chapter two were between 1998 and 2016, morbidity and mortality increased by more than 40% (Nisen, 2014). The CDC reported the problem in Reports from 1998 to 2013 titled Ten Leading Causes of Death by Age Group, Females, and The United States that showed consistency in the same top ten diseases (CDC, 1998-2013). Other notable mentions about the condition of women's health were referred to in a speech given by Dr. Bustreo of the WHO at the 2015 National Women's Day. She expressed that women's health has come a long way, but there was still a long way to go when it came to improving women's health care (WHO, 2015).

The study takes the suggestion that the position in the hospital that drives patient care and the funding for the care are health care administrators. These health care administrators are not included in many of the decisions that concern the quality of care for patients (Lagace, 2010). This is a problem for the quality of care because health care administrators help to establish the guidelines that come from the laws that are passed by state and federal government agencies (Thomas et al., 2010). The investigator interviewed ten retired health care administrators to get their input on how to develop important parameter of medical guidelines for improving the quality of women's health care. These semi-structured questions of the interviews were designed to answer the overarching reach question, "what are the relevant parameters for a medical guideline for improving the quality of women's health care?"

The chapter will start with describing the findings and conclusions of the study. Then it will move on to the limitations of the study. The next section will be the implications for practice that were uncovered in the study. The impact of the study and the recommendation for future research will be the next part of the chapter. Finally, the chapter provides a conclusion of all the information in the study.

Findings and Conclusions

The results of the survey supported that there were medical parameters in place for women's health, but there was a need for improvement in women's health care. The major themes extrapolated from this study were preventive care, education, outreach programs, and physicians' responsibility. The first two major themes were preventive care and education, and they both were being done well but still needed some improvements. The findings emphasized that preventive care and education were primary focal points for improving the quality of care for females. In the analysis of the interview responses, education was noted as not just needed for women but for medical professionals at all levels. Increased health care education was also necessary for the family members of the women so that quality health care decisions could start at home. The increase in health care education should start with children at an early age. The next theme was outreach. Developing outreach programs that can reach patients and find out why they are not coming into medical facilities before it is too late to help them was a major concern. Getting to young girls in the early stages of life to help develop good health care decisions that encourage a better quality of health and life also came out during the patient responsibility theme. The next theme was about physicians' responsibility. The responsibility is not just on doctors; their staff needs to be held responsible for providing better customer service. Customer service has to exceed the indicators on a customer service survey. Customer service needs to have compassion and empathy built into the process. There needs to be stronger consequences to consistent poor customer service complaints in the medical community. There are already several customer service programs but most of them do not have direct consequences unless the physicians own their office. Quality Assurance programs could be used to help develop programs that could assist in developing better customer service programs.

Medical responsibilities are not just a priority for physicians and their staff, but women have a responsibility to the medical professionals that care for them. They are just as responsible for the development of quality health care as any other patient. The need to change the mindset of women about their health and the importance they put on it is one of the reasons that patient responsibility was noted in the study.

The issue was that the study was looking to help develop relevant parameter guidelines that could improve the quality of health care for women. Women need to be included in the decisions concerning the laws that govern their health care and contribute to the development of improvements to their health care. Most of the laws are determined by men that do not always understand the needs of females. The responsibility to ensure patients get their preventive health care also connects to outreach programs and education. One thing that the study uncovered is the themes had a tendency to interlock and connect with each other. Preventive health care, education, and outreach programs were the primary interlocking issues. Patient-centered care was interlocked with all three major themes in the study. Some subthemes were males' part in women's health, referrals for specialty care, and the doctor-patient relationship. The results of the study were interesting and gave some important recommendations for improvements for women's health.

All the participants' responses supported the literature in Chapter Two that stated the major themes of preventive health care and education were moving in the right direction when it came to women's health but they both needed improvement (WHO, 2015). The majority of the participants stated that the major themes of outreach programs and physicians responsibility needed improvement. The literature in Chapter Two also supported this fact because it pointed out that women needed more outreach programs that could help aid women with treatment after major health events in their lives (Chase, D. M., Wenzel, L. B., & Monk, B. J. Jun 2012). The literature also stated that there was a need to improve the quality of care required in public health care (Davis, M., V., Mahanna, E., Joly, B., Zelek, M., & Riley, W., Jan 2014). The subthemes included doctor/patient relationship, male participation, specialty care, laws, and barriers to health care, quality, and technology. The connection of the subthemes and major themes are intertwined at developing action plans the support outreach. P7 made this point by stating, "what's most important is the lifestyle, what are you doing, what are you eating, how are you taking care of yourself, your rest and your exercising." . Outreach program would be used to accomplish higher educational goals for patients and health care providers. The majority of participants mentioned the need to increase community outreach where children and families lived. P4 made this point by stating, "It is almost non-existent as the Government throws women health issues into legislation packaged with the Affordable Care Act to which the current governing body is trying to repeal desperately." The cost of health care can be high but laws that can contribute to women receiving the preventive care that could detect possible issues before they become serious illnesses is crucial to developing the parameter guidelines that will improve the amount of attention that will help to improve women's health care. P6 made this point by stating, "Just get them to the door. We have first to figure out why they are not coming". The striking statement was the medical community needed to be proactive in finding out why patients were not getting the preventive care they needed. Was it because they did not have the money, they needed to pay bills instead, or maybe they had no transportation? The overall interlocking theme in question three was going out into the community with outreach services would help develop relevant parameter guidelines that would improve the quality of care for all patients', not just women.

The overall premise of the responses supported processes for helping females to develop quality mental, emotional, and physical health for themselves and their families to create a practice of wellness. The practice of wellness could follow young women into adulthood and the communities they live. Developing a system of wellness would contribute to improving the relevant parameters that would create quality care for women's health in the United States. The literature review identified the Center for Disease and Control, Institute of Medicine, and the World Health Organization as agencies that supported the themes discovered in this research study.

The first proposition of the study asserted that health care managers would be able to provide the meaningful information to contribute to defined relevant parameters of a medical guideline for improving the quality of women's health care. The participants for the semi-structured interviews were retired health care managers. They all had at least ten years' experience in the health care administrative field and lived in the Southeast. The data indicated that the administrators could contribute lots of information to the development of important parameters for a medical guideline for improving the quality of women's health care. The input they gave led to the development of four major themes. The first two themes were preventive health care and education, which they indicated were being done well but needed additional improvements. The next two major themes were outreach programs and physicians responsibility. These two themes interlocked. Both dealt with what medical professionals and the medical facilities that could do with delivering better patient health care. The subthemes to the study supported the four major themes by indicating a direction for all four major themes towards improvement and growth. The results of the study showed that health care administrators could provide information that would contribute to the development of relevant parameters of a medical guideline for improving the quality women's health care.

The second proposition of the study asserted that themes would emerge that aided in the consistency of a process for developing guidelines physicians could use to treat female patients. The administrators reflected on the issue of laws concerning women's health that were decided by men. The issue is that more women need to be at the table when the laws are being decided upon concerning women's health care. The issues with health care centered on men's health care concerns having dominance over the concerns of women's health care. Also, the need for more female physicians would help to develop the processes that would give consistency with laws and research findings and help them to be consistently transferred into relevant medical guidelines for improving the quality of women's health care. Women need to be more involved in the decisions that affect their health. They also need to take an active role in how their health care is delivered. One very relevant comment was patient-center health care. The patient is the driver, and she has the last word when it comes to deciding what will happen with her health. Getting women more involved with the decisions concerning their health care is a major step to improving the quality of their health care.

The first proposition in the study was that health care administrators/managers would be able to provide the meaningful information to contribute to the defined relevant parameters of a medical guideline for improving the quality of women's health care. The first proposition was supported with the findings because the ten retired administrators identified major themes and subthemes of processes that were being done well and areas that needed more improvement. The second proposition in the study was that themes would emerge that aided in the consistency of a process for developing guidelines physicians could use to treat female patients. There were four major themes and seven subthemes that emerged from the study and there were clear steps of improvement that were identified by the health care administrators of the study. A notable finding was that some improvements could be started immediately and some would take time, but the improvements were all achievable goals.

Limitations of the Study

In chapter one, the first limitation was life events. There were some life events in both the researchers and participants lives that caused some interviews to be rescheduled. Most were changes in schedules and life events that would come up at the last moment that caused a few reschedules for both the research and a participant. However, all ten interviews were able to be completed in the necessary timeframe.

The second limitation was a participant not wanting to participate in the study. There was only one incident where a participant did not want to take part in the study. The researcher had additional possible secondary participants, and the study was not hindered by the participant that decided not to participate in the study.

The third limitation was the possibility that a participant would not want to answer a question. No question was refused by a participant. Some participants asked for clarification, but they responded to the question once they understood what the question was asking more clearly. The limitations mentioned in Chapter one was addressed, but there was an additional barrier that occurred during the study. The investigator had no control over the participant responses. Some participants had answered questions before the question was asked. They also gave answers that the investigator did not agree with in relevance to the posed question. The researcher took all the precautions to eliminate bias demonstrated by participants, but some bias still arose in the participant responses. The way that was overcome was to focus on the similar responses made by participants. Choosing males and females to participate in the study helped to address most of the bias that came out in the research.

Implications for Practice

The study is very relevant to practitioners in the field. The points that were brought out in the study were that preventive health care and education for women concerning their health care are being done correctly but still need improvement. The consistent improvement of preventive health care and teaching is a process that practitioners can improve. As indicated in the study, classes can be started for those physicians to develop better doctor/patient relationships who did not meet the facility guidelines for patient satisfaction. Developing guidelines that are specific to female patient satisfaction will help to identify physicians and their staff that need additional compassion training through quality review. Also developing doctor/patient contracts that indicate what can be expected from the physician and what the physician expects from his or her patients is another practice that can immediately be implemented by doctors.

Other areas that could help develop better preventive care, that will take time developing, are laws like the Affordable Care Act that supports the no cost sharing preventive care service for women. The services of focus are well visits, gestational diabetes screening, human papillomavirus DNA testing, sexually transmitted infection counseling, HIV screening and counseling, contraception and contraceptive counseling, breast-feeding support, supplies and counseling, and interpersonal and domestic violence screening and counseling. These eight services start with a doctor's visit that leads to screening and testing. Additional services of focus include counseling to help support women to gain an understanding of their medical concerns and providing preventive care that is accessible and affordable to women to help women who have no health insurance get the basic preventive care and counseling that could save their lives (Sifferlin, 2012).

Education was one theme of the study that was done well. Several education programs already exist. The issue is they are not connected. If the medical community could develop a consistent a process of finding programs that could consolidate and help patients, the results could lead to the development of important parameters for developing guidelines to improve the quality of women's health care. The issue is not the educational programs that already exist but the organization of the programs. Patients may feel overwhelmed when trying to find programs that identify with their needs. The medical community could meet the needs by being more proactive in directing the patient to the right educational health organizations. The need for outreach programs is the theme from the study that will be harder to move forward. There are limitations when it comes to outreach programs. Outreach programs are an important part of education and preventive care. Several outreach programs deal with illness. Developing more outreach programs that help support wellness programs is the challenge. The United States health care system is built on caring for sick people. The United States health care system seems to prey on sick people to make money. Changing the health care system to a system of wellness is not going to be easy, but it can be done. There will have to be commitment and buy-in from both patients and medical professionals. The medical community has already started transitioning to the patient-centered care processes, but it is not a widely used practice. In addition to this, there is a need to develop programs that are centered on medical professionals becoming more empathic and compassionate when it comes to women's health care. Women need to feel comfortable with their doctors, and the additional education will also help practitioners to provide better care.

There is also a final major theme of physician responsibility. The responsibility is not just doctors; their staff needs to be held responsible for providing better customer service. Customer service has to exceed the indicators on a customer service survey. Customer service needs to have compassion and empathy built into the process. There needs to be stronger consequences to consistent poor customer service complaints in the medical community. There are already several customer service programs but most of them do not have direct consequences unless the physicians own their office. Quality Assurance programs could be used to help develop programs that could assist in developing better customer service programs.

Implications of Study and Recommendations for Future Research

There are several options for future research associated with the study findings. The need to start educating young girls about wellness early in their life is one. The suggestions are centered on teaching young girls about healthy eating habits. If they learn how to create a diet plan for themselves, it could reduce the issues in the United States concerning obesity. Three participants made several comments about diet, exercise, and obesity.

Lower-income families need to learn how they can afford the foods that would help develop the eating habits that could help decrease many of the health issues found on the CDC list of Ten Disease of Morbidity and Mortality in Women of All Ages in the United States. The top ten diseases were heart disease, stroke, chronic lower respiratory, and COPD, which all fall under cardiovascular disease. It also listed cancer, Alzheimer's, influenza and pneumonia, kidney disease, Septicemia, and Diabetes (CDC, 1998-2013). Many of these diseases are hereditary, but this does not mean that a woman has to develop them. Also if patients develop the diseases found on the CDC listing, they may not be as severe as they would be if they are on a healthy diet. The other benefit of teaching young girls to develop healthy life habits is the advantage to the family. The outreach programs and the teaching of proper diet, exercise, and wellness could be translated into healthy families with good life habits. Many programs are said to be following this pattern, but there needs to be a scale that would determine the effectiveness of these programs. Processes that evaluate programs educating young girls about healthy eating and how to make better life decisions may help to develop important parameters that would improve the quality of health care

The second recommendation was the concern about doctors developing relationships with their patients. The training should go beyond compassion training. Compassion training is being done, but there is still an issue with the doctor/patient relationship as it relates to women patients. Many of the participants had stories about not feeling heard by their doctors. Some of those participants were men who were not happy with the care that a female family member received. Most of the concerns and comments were directly related to the doctor/patient relationship. An introduction to more than compassion training into the medical system could be the way ahead for building a better doctor/patient relationship with women patients. One participant commented that it is not just about empathy and compassion but about customer service. It was that participant's belief that the quality of care in the United States was good, but the customer service was what was lacking. Developing a program that is designed specifically for developing empathy, compassion, and customer service for female patients would be different from what is being done presently. The medical community is starting to look at women differently because of the high mortality and morbidity rates. The suggestion could be similar to the outreach programs. To develop a program that determined the effectiveness of programs that already exist as it relates to women patients would be a good qualitative study that could be done on the perception of female patients and how they relate to their doctors. The specific direction of the study would be to address issues that outline possible training programs that could address the issue of doctor/patient relationship.

Another problem noted in the study was how improving women's health care could improve the health care of all patients. The outreach programs suggestion was closely tied to the suggested future study. When looking at all these proposals, there is a pattern of there being other studies that have been done. The issue is not that studies have not been done and results have not been valid the problem is that this is where the studies stopped. Study results need to have action plans, or they need to be translated into guidelines that can be used in field women's health care. Conducting a study that helps develop consistent evaluation processes that test the efficiency and effectiveness of how study results are translated and used is another future study suggestion.

There was mention about over saturation of male involvement with laws that are passed concerning women's health care. As noted in other studies that were summarized in the literature review (Cambronero-Saiz, 2013), the problem was not the development of outreach programs. The problem was the effectiveness of outreach programs. Part of the issue is how much women want to be involved in their health care. Women do care about their health, but the need for them to take care of their families and work responsibilities takes priority over their health care. Once women start campaigning for the positions that put them in the place where they can decide legislation, then women can get seats at the table and their voices can be heard. There are statistical studies about the issue, but there need to be programs that encourage young girls and women to develop the skills that will put them in the positions of power that decides on legislation.

Many of the suggestions surround programs that have been started. The suggested concern of this study is how effective are the existing programs. There is no need to start new programs until the effectiveness of existing programs is reviewed and corrected to achieve the desired goal of the program. Other areas of concern are outreach programs that will develop a system in early childhood to educate young girls. These programs would encourage young girls to be more focused on education, proper eating habits, proper exercise, and healthy life habits. Being pretty is nice but being healthy, being educated, and making good life decisions it more important. The future of women's health is centered on teaching wellness. Programs are needed that encourage women to make the health decisions that are needed to develop a quality life that will support quality health care for them and their families. Women need to take responsibility for their part in the lack of quality concerning their health care. They have a tendency to make the decision based on the needs of their friends and families. They also need to start showing an active presence when it comes to developing the laws that concern their health care. In addition to women's responsibility, medical professionals have a responsibility to ensure their patients are provided quality care. The health care system needs to be actively involved in recruiting quality female doctors to help care for women. This recruitment process is crucial when changing the quality of health care for females. It is not that outreach programs have not been started and that recruiting efforts have not been started; it is that these issues need to be improved when it comes to women's health.

Conclusion

The purpose of this explorative qualitative study was to discover relevant parameters of medical guidelines for improving the quality of women's health care. The study suggested by both the literature and the interviews of the participants that there was a need to improve the quality of care for women's health. The study did point out that there were areas that were being done correctly by the medical professionals. Even with this thought process the literature and the participants suggested that there was still a need to improve areas of women's health care.

The overarching question of the study was, "what are the relevant parameters for a medical guideline for improving the quality of women's health care?" The overarching suggestion to the question was teaching wellness to both patients and doctors. The major themes of the study were preventive health care, education, outreach programs, and physician's responsibility. The subthemes were doctor/patient relationship, male participation, specialty care, laws, barriers to health care, quality, technology, patient-center health care. The subthemes supported the major themes.

The health care administrators that participated in the study demonstrated responses that were completely supportive of the literature in Chapter 2 of the study. Their responses also supported the purpose statement of the study that was to discover the relevant parameters of a medical guideline for improving the quality of women's health care was achievable. The results of the study answered the overarching question of, "what are the relevant parameters for a medical guideline for improving the quality of women's health care? Health care administrators could develop programs that surrounded the development of outreach programs that would increase the effectiveness of preventive health care by meeting women patients in their environment. Going into the environment would include programs that find out what patients need to ensure they get the preventive services and examines. Also by developing educational outreach programs that teach healthy diet, exercise, and developing skills that will help women patients, the process could assist young women to learn how to choose healthier life decisions at a young age. In addition to developing outreach programs for preventive health care and education, there should also be programs that help with providing preventive health services at an affordable cost. The next step in the process would be to ensure that physicians take responsibility for the success of these programs and develop the types of relationships that would create teamwork between them and their patients.

Other possible improvements was the development of programs that dealt with the effectiveness of preventive health care, education, outreach programs, and physician's responsibility as it related to women's health care. Several existing programs have focused on all the major themes. The issue is, as stated in the literature, that the results of many of the studies and programs have not been translated into effective guidelines that could improve the quality of care women receive. One of the participants did not think the quality of care was poor, she believed that the issue is poor customer service. It is about how women were made to feel when it came to their health care by medical professionals. Women need to feel like they are heard and that their concerns are important. Outreach programs that help all medical professionals and medical staff go out into the community and find out why patients are not coming in for preventive health care and that educate by teaching proper diet, exercise, and healthy life decisions were other suggestions.

The key finding in the study centered on developing effectiveness. All the programs and themes have been investigated, and programs have been started, but women's mortality and morbidity rates still climbed to over 40% between 1998 and 2013 (Nisen, 2011). Just having a program is not enough. Just doing a study is not sufficient. Studies need action plans and translation into guidelines that can support increased quality of health care for women.

The ten health care administrators stressed, as the study stated, that if they were not excluded from the initial decision process, improvements would not take so long to be put into action. The health care administrators asserted that women needed to be more involved in the decisions that affected the laws that surrounded their health care. Health care is male driven, and women need to be more proactive about being at the decision tables that involve legislation and decisions that affect their health care. The process of developing programs that encourage involvement of women takes time, but the process needs to be started to achieve the desired goal for decreased mortality and morbidity in women's health.

References

"About Go Red" (2016). Retrieved on April 25, 2016, retrieved from https://www.goreadforwomen.org/home/about-go-red/.

"Affordable Care Act Rules on Expanding Access to Preventive Services for Women" (2016). Retrieved on April 7, 2016, retrieved on http://www.hhs.gov/healthcare/facts-and-features/fact-sheets/aca-rules-on-expanding-acces.

Bailey, M. & DiPrete, T., Issue and Conference on "The Changing Roles and Status of Women and Effects on Society and Economy" (2016). Retrieved on May 12, 2016, retrieved from https://www.russellsage.org/publications/category/current_rfa_rsfjournal/women_society.

Brown, J., Kobbler, P., & Lutzus, L. (Producers), Glatzer, R. & Westmoreland, W., *Still Alice*, Sony Pictures Classics, Kiler Films (2014).

Bruce, J., "6 Reasons Women Still Aren't Getting Paid What They Deserve," *Forbes* (May 13, 2016). Retrieved on May 18, 2016, retrieved from http://www.forbes.com/sites/janbruce/2016/05/13/6-reasons-women-still-arent-getting-pai...

Bustreo, F., Dr., "Promoting health through the life-course, ten top issues for women's health" (2015). Retrieved on June 18, 2015, retrieved from http://www.who.int/life-course/news/2015-intl-womens-day/en/.

Caiazza, A., Shaw, A., & Werschkul, M., "The Status of Women in the States, Women's Economic Status in the States: Wide Disparities by Race, Ethnicity, and Region," Institute for Women's Policy Research, Washington, DC (2016).

Cillizza, C., "Hillary Clinton May Not Recover from Her Pneumonia Until Late October" (Sep 2013). Retrieved on Sep 16, 2016, retrieved from https://www.washingtonpost.com/news/the-fix/wp/2016/09/13/it-could-take-hillary-clinton.

Courtney, V., *The Virtuous Women, Shattering the Superwoman Myth*, LifeWay Press (2000), Nashville, TN 37234-0151.

Definition of Doctor, Norton Safe Search (2016). Retrieved on Aug 22, 2016, retrieved from https://nortonsafe.search.ask.com/web?q=Definition+of+doctor&chn=&geo=en_US&o=A.

Definition of Economics, Norton Safe Search (2016). Retrieved on Aug 22, 2016, retrieved from https://nortonsafe.search.ask..com/web?q-definition+of+economic&chn=&geo-en_US&o.

Definition Health Care, Merriam-Webster (2016). Retrieved on Aug 22, 2016, retrieved from http://www.merriam-webster.com/dictionary/health%20care.

Definition of Morbidity, Merriam Webster (2016). Retrieved on Aug 22, 2016, retrieved from http://www.merriam-webster.com/dictionary/morbidity.

Definition of Nursing, ICN 1987 (2016). Retrieved on Aug 22, 2016, retrieved from http://www.icn.ch/who-we-are/icn-definition-of-nursing/.

Definition of Sociology, Merriam Webster (2016). Retrieved on Aug 22, 2016, retrieved from http://www.merriam-webster.com/dictionary/sociology.

Definition of Standard of Care, (2016), Medicinenet.com. Retrieved on Aug 22, 2016, retrieved from http://www.medicine-net.com/script/main/art.asp?articlekey=33263&pf=2.

Di Venere, L., (Sep 1, 2012), "Women's Health Under the Affordable Care Act: What is Covered?" *The Journal of Family Practice*. Retrieved on May 4, 2016, retrieved from http://www.jfponline.com/print-friendly/womens-health-under-the-affordable-care-act.

The Dr. Oz Show (2016). Retrieved on Oct 24, 2016, retrieved from http://www.doctoroz.com/

England, P., Final Report of the Committee on the Status of Women (May 21, 2009). Retrieved on May 12, 2016.

"Fact Sheet: Women & Socioeconomic Status, American Psychology Association." Retrieved on May 12, 2016, retrieved from http://www.apa.org/print-this.aspx.

Giddens, Anthony, Duneier, M., Applebaum, R., & Carr, D., "Gender Inequality," Chapter 10, Chapter Study Outline, *Introduction to Sociology*, 8th Edition, W.W. Norton & Company Inc. (2011). Retrieved on May 12, 2016, retrieved from http://www.wwnorton.com/college/soc/introductionsociology8/ch/10/outline.aspx.

Helfrich, C.A., & Simpson, E. K., "Improving Services for Lesbian Clients: What Do Domestic Violence Agencies Need to Do? Health Care for Women International" (2006), 27:344-361.

Nashawaty, C., "Still Alice" (Jan 23, 2015). Retrieved on April 25, 2016, retrieved from EW.com.

Patient Protection and Affordable Care Act (2016). Retrieved on Aug 22, 2016, retrieved from https://www.healthinsurance.org/glossary/patient-protection-and-affordable-care-act-ppaca/.

Perz, J. & Ussher, J. M., "Women's experience of premenstrual syndrome: a case of silencing the self," *Journal of Reproduction and Infant Psychology*, Vol. 24, No. 4 (Nov 2006), pp.289-303.

Perry, T., "Madea's Big Happy Family," *Entertainment Weekly*, Issue 1138 (Jan 21, 2001), p 46

"Phenomenology," Stanford Encyclopedia of Philosophy (2016). Retrieved on June 6, 2016, retrieved from http://plato.stanford.edu/entries/phenomenology/.

"Qualitative Research Terms and Definitions" (2016). Retrieved on June 6, 2016, retrieved from https://www2.med.psu.edu/humanities/research/qualitative-research-terms-and-definitions/.

Salganicoff, A., Ranji, U., Beamesderfer, A., & Kurani, N., "Women and Health Care in the Early Years of the ACA: Key Findings from the 2013 Kaiser Women's Health Survey" (May 15, 2014). Retrieved on April 27, 2016, retrieved from http://kff.org/women-health-policy/report/women-and-health-care-in-the-early-years-of-th.

Sebelius, K., Report to Congress, "Report on Activities Related to 'Improving Women's Health' As Required by the Affordable Care Act," P.L. 111-148, Section 3509 (March 23, 2011).

U.S. Department of Health and Human Services Office of the Secretary Office of the Assistant Secretary for Health Office on Women's Health.

Sedlak, C. A., Doheny, M. O., Estok, P. J., & Zeller, R. A., "Alcohol Use in Women 65 Years of Age and Older, Health Care for Women International," 21:567-581 (2000).

Sifferlin, A., "The 8 Preventive Health Services that Women Start Getting Free Today" (Aug 1, 2012). Retrieved on April 27, 2016, retrieved from http://healthland.time.com/2012/08/01/the-8-preventive-health-services-that-women-start-.

"Ten Leading Causes of Death by Age Group, Females- United States, 1998-2014," HHS, CDC, NCHS. Retrieved on April 25, 2016, retrieved from http://www.cdc.gov/nchs/dealth.htm.

"What Do Hospital Health Care Managers Do?" (2016). Retrieved on April 27, 2016, retrieved from http://programs.online

.utica.edu/articles/what-do-hospital-health-care-managers-do.asp.

"What is a Clinical Manager in Healthcare Administration?" (2016). Retrieved on April 27, 2016, retrieved from http://www.healthcare-administratin-degree.net/faq/1036-2.

"What Does a Health Care Manager Do?" (2016), Learn.org. Retrieved on Aug 22, 2016, retrieved from http://learn.org/articles/What_Does_a_Health_Care_Manager_do.html.

"What is quality of life?" (2016), Concept, HRQOL, CDC. Retrieved on Aug 22, 2016, retrieved from http://www.cdc.gov/hrqol/concept.htm.

"Why the Affordable Care Act Matters for Women: Restriction on Abortion Coverage," National Partnership for Women & Families (Mar 2002), 1875 Connecticut Avenue, NW, Suite 650, Washington, DC 20009. Retrieved on April 27, 2016, retrieved from www.NationalPartnership.org.

"Women and the Economics of Equality" *Harvard Business Review*, Economics (April 2013). Retrieved on May 18, 2016, retrieved from https://hbr.org/2013/04/women-and-the-economics-of-equality.

Women's Cancer Fund, Remembrance Run, Traverse City Track Club (2016). Retrieved on April 25, 2016, retrieved from www.munsonhealthcare.org/foundation.

Zamora, D., "Women's Top 5 Health Concerns: From heart disease to breast cancer to Depression, WebMD gives you the inside info on why women are at risk for these problems but may not know it" (2015). Retrieved on June 18, 2015, retrieved from http://www.webmd.com/women/features/5-top-female-health-concerns.